It's not over till the Bag Lady rings

howto books

Please send for a free copy of the latest catalogue:
How To Books
Spring Hill House, Spring Hill Road,
Begbroke, Oxford OX5 1RX, United Kingdom
info@howtobooks.co.uk
www.howtobooks.co.uk

Ian F. Spratley

It's not over till the Bag Lady rings

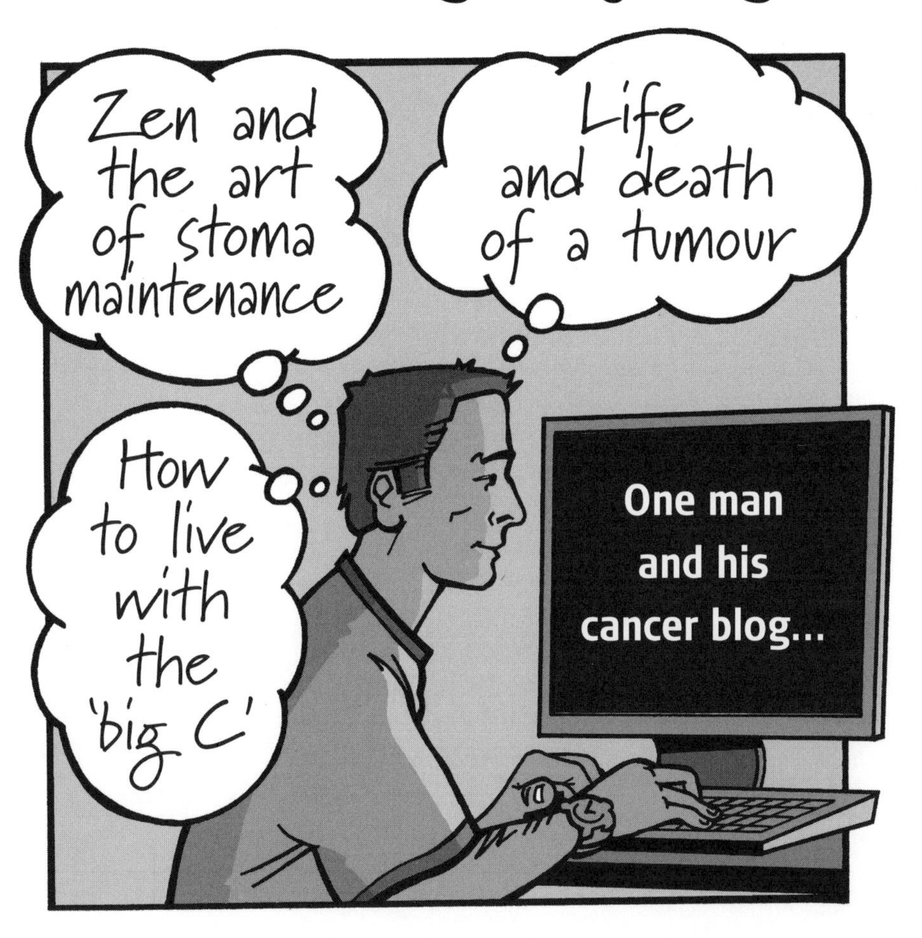

howtobooks

Published by Spring Hill

Spring Hill is an imprint of
How To Books Ltd
Spring Hill House, Spring Hill Road,
Begbroke, Oxford OX5 1RX, United Kingdom
Tel: (01865) 375794 Fax: (01865) 379162
info@howtobooks.co.uk
www.howtobooks.co.uk

British Library Cataloguing in Publication Data
A catalogue record for this book is available from
the British Library.

First published 2007

ISBN: 978 1 905862 14 6

Text and cover illustrations by David Mostyn
Produced for Spring Hill Books by Deer Park Productions, Tavistock
Typeset by *specialist* publishing services ltd, Montgomery
Printed and bound by Cromwell Press, Trowbridge, Wiltshire

Contents

ACKNOWLEDGEMENTS

Teresa Williams at MK Hospital for doing what no-one else dares.
Vanessa Cook at MK Hospital for constant reassurance.
Mr Talib Al-Mishlab and his team at MK Hospital for their surgical skills.
Neil Mercer for encouraging me to write.
Al, Alan, Bob, Cavan, Chris, Dave, Gaye, Helen, Hilary, Irene, Ian D, Ian E, Jenny, John, Karin, Lyn, Margaret, Marion, Nicola, Pauline, Pete, Rachel, Sarah, Steve, Tim, Chris K, Dan and Emma for being there.
Fat Freddy's Cat for keeping the microphone warm.
The Faculty of Education and Language Studies at the Open University for keeping my desk warm.
Giles and Nikki at Spring Hill Books for believing in the book.
Nick and Maureen at *specialist* publishing services for editorial advice and the selection of comments.
All the people who commented on my blog – friends and strangers alike.
All the people in MK, Northampton and the Oxford Hospitals – staff and patients – who gave me the time of day.
Annie – for never complaining. For always putting me first, no matter how bad she was feeling. I really don't know how I would have got through this without her.

For Annie

and

all those hurt by this wretched disease

INTRODUCTION

In the beginning there was diagnosis. And diagnosis begat phone call and phone call begat email and email begat blog and blog begat book.

I wrote the blog [a] that forms the basis of this book for a variety of reasons – initially to keep me sane, but ultimately because I want you (whoever you are and where ever you might be) to know how it *feels* to have cancer. Cancer affects the mind as well as the body.

You may already know, of course, and perhaps we can just compare notes. But many people don't. There is plenty of information out there about the mechanics of cancer – drugs, treatments, surgery and so on. But nothing I read could really prepare me for how this wretched disease would make me *feel*. Having to deal with the bits they don't tell you about – the big stuff – like confronting your own mortality, or the more prosaic – like not having clothes that fit anymore; like stoma bags that leak in the middle of the night; or simply wanting to run away and hide.

Of course this is just my experience – and many people experience it in different ways. But, judging by the emails and comments left on my blog, some parts have struck a chord with others.

Hi Ian, it's quite a relief to be able to talk to someone who is experiencing almost the same as me!

Heather, 11th September 2006

I never expected to write a book – or rather have my blog published in this form. I simply started using email as a means of keeping in touch with friends and family – just progress reports to begin with – then a few anecdotes about my stay in hospital first time round. I decided to include the grim bits and the mucky bits as well as the comic bits. It wouldn't be cancer without the dark side, but I did see a funny side as well. Hospitals are ripe for story-telling – the dramatic and the ridiculous side by side.

Nurses are very funny people – I guess they have to be – and if they can laugh at it so can I. If I didn't laugh, I'd cry. And I did cry. But not all the time.

The response to my emails was staggering – friends, acquaintances – people I hadn't seen in years – all got in touch and offered support – from practical help to simply listening. Some friends passed my emails on to others – people they knew who were also affected by this disease. Suddenly email became too limiting – I wanted to tell the world how I felt and so decided to keep an on-line diary – a blog.

A blog, unlike email, is a bit like a message in a bottle – it's not aimed at anyone in particular – it's just a matter of writing and tossing it into the ocean. Would anyone find it? I wasn't sure, but the simple act of writing allowed me to think that someone out there was listening.

In the event it washed up on a number of people's computers and strangers from around the world took time to write to me – either leaving comments on the blog or by email. I felt uplifted by the love and warmth of all these strangers – I was crowd surfing in the cancer mosh pit [b].

I started to enjoy the process of setting out my thoughts – sometimes nothing more than a record of events, at other times a stream of consciousness-type ramble – because as I looked back at what I had written, it seemed as if the cancer was moving from me to the page (or screen if you're a pedant). Word by word it made *me* feel better. Then one day I received the following email from a woman in Malaysia:

I almost gave up on the bag when it leaked every day … When I read your diary, it made me feel that we are not alone… Somewhere at the other side of the world someone understands my situation… That's really made me relieved… Thanks… Ocean of love.

Julie, 24th July 2006

I had not realised others were going through the same thing as me. That's part of the trouble with cancer – it can make you very self-centred. I wondered how this woman had found me. It turns out she had simply entered 'stoma bag leakage' into Google and arrived at my blog. (I tried *Googling* 'stoma bag leakage' and gave up after 30 pages – I guess she was just lucky – or persistent). We to and fro'd about leaking bags, bag design and just the sheer hell of dealing with this stuff.

I got other emails and comments; some from people who had been through it all and had come out the other side, some who were going through it and some from people who were carers, loved ones or friends of cancer patients. A few defied classification – they simply wished me well, without leaving a clue as to their own situation: The kindness of strangers.

Some people relived their own experience of the disease – they saw my progress and could look back at their own and see how far they had come. Others simply found it a help in getting through their own suffering. I received one email from someone in the Personnel Department of a large organisation. She said that cases for sick leave for people with cancer often landed on her desk, but until she read the blog, she had no idea what it *felt* like to have this disease. Result.

I've included some of these comments in this book to show the generosity and insight of others. Most of the emails have been deleted because I didn't think to keep them – because I didn't expect to publish the blog ...

This book covers the period from diagnosis in December 2005 to just beyond the first anniversary of that diagnosis. Although it takes the form of a diary it has a narrative structure – there is a beginning, a middle and an end – of sorts.

My hope is that, by reading this account, you'll have a better understanding of what cancer patients have to deal with (if you don't already know) or, if you do know, you can say '*Yeah – been there, done that, got the tee-shirt – and lived to tell the tale*'.

My hope in writing is that the pain and discomfort and fear that I've been through in the past year or so will not have been for nothing – that something positive and tangible will come out of the experience. Writing has become synonymous with my cancer and it's as if when I hold the book in my hand the cancer is out there in the world – and not in me.

A quick search on *Amazon* will reveal a lot of books on cancer – many like this. So who is mine aimed at? When I started writing I wanted to inform friends and family; then I wanted to inform others – patients, carers and healthcare professionals – anyone who'd listen. A tall order perhaps. As far as I'm concerned it's a rung in the ladder of understanding. The best sales pitch came in an email from someone who cares for cancer patients:

Your personal contribution will represent a very valuable piece of literature on every library shelf – and I am asking that it is listed on the required reading list for all my friends, patients, staff and clinical colleagues.

Barbara, 27th January 2007

Looking back I find it hard to recognise myself. I know it's about me, but I can't remember all the pain and discomfort and fear that I experienced. Part of me doesn't want to – but another part does. If I forget the effect it had on me I'll forget the effect it had – or has – on others. And I don't want to do that.

At the time of writing this Introduction (February 2007) my prognosis is 'guarded'. Cancer is a disease we should know so much about, because it's so common. But we don't – each time a discovery increases our understanding, cancer cheats to get back in the game: like bowel cancer cells which play dead to avoid getting zapped by chemo drugs. But my outlook remains positive. Treatments *are* improving all the time and I am determined to be one of the lucky ones.

I know it's a cliché but this disease has changed my life forever. The hardest thing for me is living in a permanent state of uncertainty. Doctors never say the word 'cure'. The further away I get from first diagnosis the better the chances of survival. It's always about numbers. I guess though, living with uncertainty is a rather good problem to have. At least it's living.

[a] Blog: an on-line diary. From We**b log**.
[b] Ask any teenager who's interested in music.

THE DIARY

A very important earache

Late December 2005

The run up to Christmas was dismal as far as I was concerned. Goodwill to all men was hard to muster; it was more a case of '*bah rock cake*' than '*bah humbug*'. (This reference to the baker's art will be explained shortly).

When I first discovered I had cancer – coming out of sedation after an colonoscopy – I managed to get over the shock and fear by simply being positive. I now realise that it's very easy to confuse positive thinking with naïvety.

The hospital gave me an information pack to take home; a description of the operation, a colostomy bag to play with and a brochure with photographs of happy, smiling people getting on with their lives. I glanced through the short, and to the point, leaflet entitled 'lower anterior resection', the crude but effective diagrams helping what was about to happen to sink in. I couldn't bear to touch the colostomy bag or read about happy people.

I decided I needed to tell people about this. I started firing off emails – I found it easier to write than telephone – in the hope that someone I knew was bound to know someone who had gone through this and survived. I needed positive stories from real people, rather than manufactured ones – I was quite capable of providing the alternative scenarios myself. Sure enough my optimism was rewarded. I was inundated with tales of 80-year-olds leaping off mountains and bike riders with bags under their Lycra® (the mind – and the shorts – boggle).

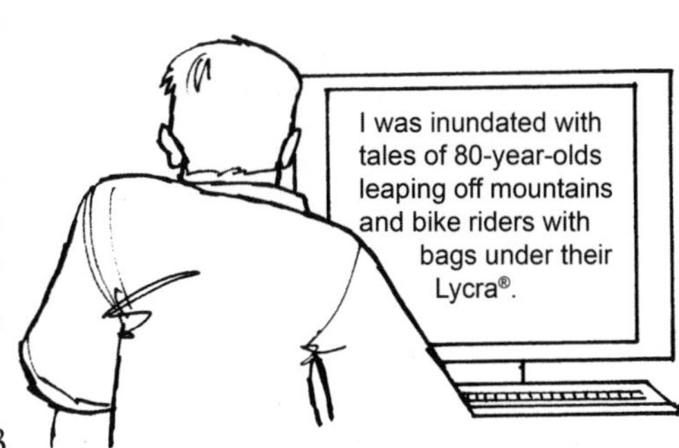

I really began to think that this was no big deal and saw it as no more than an inconvenience. It was turning out to be so common. Which is frightening, as well as reassuring, when you think about it. My good spirits lasted precisely a week. I was devastated when I discovered that the cancer had spread to my liver. This was now serious. I sunk into depression – a state of mind compounded by everything I read. The NHS Direct website suggests that once the cancer cells have spread to the liver, the disease is usually 'incurable'. It may be controlled for some years though. A chill went through my body as I read these words.

Someone said, '*You must be angry*'. I realised I was not – I simply felt an overwhelming sadness. I was extremely happy with my lot; the children were getting on with their lives, I was playing in a fantastic band[1] and Annie and I were setting out on a new life together. Now I began to wonder what sort of life that would be. She didn't deserve this.

The turning point came on Christmas day. Not feeling like being sociable, I sat on the bed alone reading Alan Bennett's '*Untold Stories'*. To my great surprise and delight, it included an essay about his bowel cancer – '*An Average Size Rock Cake'* – a reference to his surgeon's description of his tumour. Here was a first-hand account by someone who had faced the same fears and gently, through a mix of humour and uncompromising honesty, lead me to understand what to expect in a way that the internet and the leaflets, written by healthcare professionals – no matter how well intentioned – could never do.

He even had his own 'chilling' moment. Nick Leeson (*Barings Bank*) developed bowel cancer while in jail. This was a big story and media interest was intense. A reporter asked a doctor what would happen if it spread to his liver: '*He's a dead man*'. Bennett wondered what effect that bit of news would have on bowel cancer sufferers around the world. He's been in remission for over five years and concludes his essay with *'take heart'*. Which I did.

I spoke to the colorectal nurse at the hospital about how I was feeling. She said that the idea that cancer cells in the liver meant the disease was untreatable was at least five years out of date. She advised care when looking up health websites. I resolved not to read any more 'official' literature on bowel cancer. I'd had enough. Words can just fly off the page and crash land.

I also realised how lucky I had been to have had earache in November. This came at the end of almost two weeks of constant diarrhoea. I don't think these two events are related. The band had played a gig in Leicester and we all went out for an Indian meal afterwards. At first I put my upset stomach down to this and didn't think too much of it. Annie also had a stomach bug at the same time, so I might have caught that. After about ten days it started to ease, only to be replaced by earache. It got so bad that I went to see my GP about it. Having sorted it out I mentioned, almost in passing, the diarrhoea. He did a quick examination and referred me at once to a colorectal consultant. I was seen within two weeks, had cancer confirmed within another two weeks and had surgery a month later. Pretty good going. Like the man said – take heart.

[1] Fat Freddy's Cat; an acoustic, tex-mex, soul-grass, whatever you want to call it, band. See *www.fatfreddyscat.com*

A new bike

Early January 2006

I bought a new bike about a week before the operation. It was a completely spur of the moment thing – I surprised myself as much as the bike shop owner. I had intended to buy a new bike in a few months' time – after the operation as a spur to recovery, a treat – something to lighten the dark days ahead.

But I found myself driving past the bike shop this particular morning and decided to drop in. I've always found bike shops fascinating places to while away a few minutes. Whenever I visit a new town, at home or abroad, I always seek out the local bike shop. Some people head for bookshops, others museums. I kill time in the bike shop. There's always something to see or someone to chat to.

My motives were mixed this time; it was January and I was looking forward to the summer, so a quick look through the new season's clothing was on the agenda. But I also hoped the owner would be around. I knew he had been ill and I wanted another positive story to keep me going. I was in luck – he was there. We chatted about his cancer, my cancer, the NHS, our families, the things we had been prepared for and the things that had taken us by surprise. We eventually got round to bikes and I mentioned that I would be ordering a new one once I was in recovery, but I was unsure about the size. He had one in the workshop I could try. I was in luck again. It turned out to be the previous year's model – a much nicer colour scheme in my view than the one I had originally set my sights on.

I rode it up and down the road and thought about the summer in France where Annie and I had spent an idyllic two weeks with our bikes. This was the part I could not understand; I was fit and healthy. I was happy. I eat a good balanced diet (at least five fruit and vegetables a day) and I'm riding a bike. And – according to the hospital staff – when I come out of hospital in about ten days' time, my leg muscles will have gone and I'll need someone to fetch and carry for me. In other words, I'm going to come out of hospital a lot worse than when I went in. It just didn't make sense.

The bike was perfect and when I got back to the shop I spent a while just looking at it, lost in my own world. Was I really going to be able to ride a bike again? I heard from someone who had taken six months to get to the stage where he could ride just ten miles. But people do get over bowel cancer, even when it has spread to the liver. The shop owner broke the mood – he offered me 20% discount (a not inconsiderable sum), as it was last year's model. This was utter madness. Do I really need a new bike now? What if the operation goes wrong – would Annie be able to sell it? I looked at the bike again as my credit card lay on the counter.

As I wheeled it from the shop the owner said '*I hope you get some miles from it*'. It was the way he said '*some*' that made me realise that something unspoken had passed between us. We both knew I might not.

The Homer Simpson diet

Early January 2006

I'm impressed by the support I'm getting from the hospital. I have two nurses from a multi-disciplinary team that I can talk to; Vanessa (a colorectal specialist) who deals with the cancer and its treatment and Teresa (a stoma care specialist – The Bag Lady) who will teach me to empty, clean and change the bag – or pouch as it is more properly called – when I come out of hospital.

Vanessa had already explained that because the cancer is low down in the bowel there was a chance that they might not be able to simply cut out the offending part and join the two healthy ends together. Even if they could, the join would need time to heal so either way I would need to have a stoma – an opening in the stomach wall – to get rid of waste materials while the bowel was unable to function. If a join were possible, I would have a temporary ileostomy with a bag attached to the small colon (ileum). If a join were not possible I would have a permanent colostomy, with a bag attached to the large colon. The consensus was that a join would be the more likely outcome so I should expect an ileostomy – but be prepared for a colostomy.

For me at least, the difference between the two is far, far greater than simply being temporary or permanent. That's not to say one is worse than the other, they are both life changing and each has its own unique set of challenges. I am squeamish at the best of times and am not looking forward to either. The ileostomy offers hope that it may be temporary – perhaps a year, rather than having to deal with this for the rest of my life. It's the position of the ileostomy that presents me with a particular challenge.

Losing a chunk of bowel means there is less available for food processing. So it's likely that I will have to give up nuts and corn, which turn out to be the most difficult foods to break down. In most colostomies some of the large bowel, where fibre is broken down, will still function so it's possible to have a reasonably balanced diet. But the ileostomy is attached to the small colon, bypassing the large bowel altogether. With no large bowel, I cannot process fibre. And in order to recover from surgery I'll have to greatly increase my intake of protein and fat.

As someone who is used to eating a healthy diet this comes as a bit of a shock and means I will have to change my eating habits for a while. I talk it over with the Bag Lady: no fibre, fibre is dangerous as the strands can accrete and form a blockage. So, no citrus fruits, no wholemeal bread, rice, nuts, seeds, berries, broccoli, pulses – in fact all the things I love and eat regularly. I will also lose a lot of salt because the output from the stoma will be diluted. So, I'll need to add salt to my meals (which I never do) and eat plenty of crisps and cheese and biscuits. And white bread. And white rice. And chips. And pizza. And meat – because I need the protein and can't get it from pulses. The ideal meal appears to be burger and chips followed by a doughnut for dessert. The unhealthiest part is the sesame seeds on the bun ... The cure for bowel cancer appears to be a heart attack.

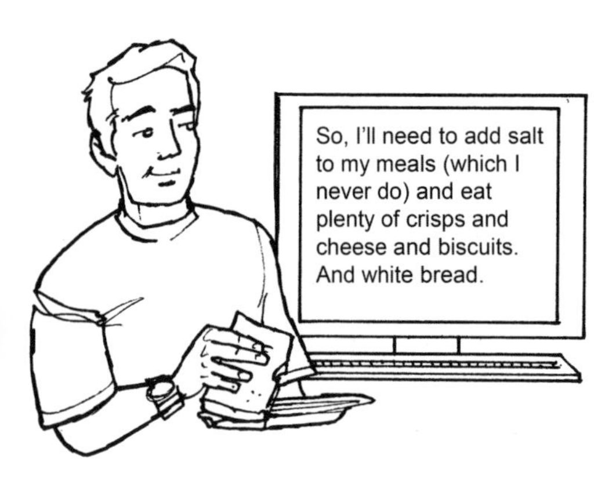

The Jolly Green Giant

Mid January 2006

Hospital can be a lonely place. Although there are nurses, other patients and visitors, most of the time is spent in isolation. Sometimes this can make a welcome change from a busy life, but at other times the ward just seems to be full of men sitting in chairs beside their beds staring into space. The isolation does not seem to be either welcome or profitable.

The loneliest time, for me at least, is the night before the operation.

Visiting time is over and Annie has gone. A steady stream of medical staff only serves to increase the sense of loneliness; first a doctor to take a blood sample, then the Bag Lady to draw the spot on my belly for the stoma. In fact she draws two spots – one on the left in case I have a colostomy and one on the right in case it's an ileostomy. This uncertainty only adds to my apprehension. An anaesthetist comes to discuss 'pain management' and finally a surgeon arrives with a consent form. He's a big man, always laughing and by his accent I assume him to be African.

Having spent the past six hours getting through four litres of *Kleen-Prep* (a form of liquid drain unblocker) I am not best able to concentrate. He shows me the form, drawing my attention to the side effects. Most are scribbled and I can't make out the writing, but in capital letters he's written 'DEATH'. The whole business of consent seems ridiculous at this stage. I have cancer and I'm about to have – what is, everyone tells me – a routine operation to remove it:

'We would not put you through this if we did not think the prognosis was good.'

How can I withdraw my consent at this stage? I'm not comparing like with like. Surely the cancer is considerably more life threatening than the operation? I sign the form. But as I'm about to find out, the cancer and the operation are pretty evenly matched.

I wake early next morning and take a bath as requested. I've had nothing to eat for 36 hours now. By 8.45am I'm on my way to theatre. Annie will be teaching by now. I hope she's OK. If this were an episode of *Casualty* or *Holby City*, she'd be here while I'm wheeled down to theatre. It's Friday 13th. Should I be worried?

The theatre staff are welcoming and reassuring. A nurse holds my hand while they explain in great detail what they're going to do. I wonder if she does this for every patient or does she sense my unease? The end result will be a general anaesthetic, but the process starts with more gentle sedation so they can insert an epidural. The drugs take effect and I relax and let them do what they have to do.

They've almost finished when The Jolly Green Giant appears. It's the surgeon from the night before. He's in scrubs and a mask but I recognise the laugh: *'I hope you got a big pelvis so I can get these big hands in'*.

He waves a pair of enormous fists in my face. I suddenly remember one of the side effects of the operation. They will have to move the pelvic nerves to get at the large bowel. If the nerves are damaged or severed my sex life will be seriously compromised – perhaps permanently. I remember thinking *'oh ****'* then *zzzzzzzz-zzzzzzzzzzzzzzzzzzz.*

Houston – we have a problem

Mid January 2006

I woke from surgery feeling very cold. And completely numb from the waist down. I was wrapped in blankets to get my temperature up. I could hear voices – I could make out my name being called, but not much else. I have no idea how long I was in recovery for – I dozed off again and woke up in the ward. Annie was there. I guessed it was Friday evening, but I'm not sure.

The consultant came to see me. The operation had gone so well that they had decided not to give me a stoma. I was bag-less. I couldn't believe it – this was just wonderful news.

By Saturday the tube had been removed from my throat and I could sit up in bed. The tube had made my throat sore and talking was difficult – my voice had dropped and Annie thought I should start adding Tom Waits' songs to my repertoire. By visiting time in the afternoon, I was planning to sit in on a gig scheduled for the end of the month. It all seemed possible.

Monday evening I had pins and needles in my right hand and arm.

My heart rate started racing. I had a suspected *'abnormal heart arrhythmia'*. Over the coming days I began to feel unwell and my stomach swelled to *Michelin Man* proportions. The consensus was that whatever had happened on the Monday night had meant that the blood supply to the join had been cut off and it had developed a leak. A decision was made to take me back into theatre for an ileostomy to take pressure off the join. A second major operation in a week. I was past caring – I just wanted to feel better.

The man who mistook a lamp for a penguin

Mid January 2006

The pain management afforded by the epidural was very effective. I could control how and when I needed pain killers through the use of a small hand-held release. The effectiveness of this system was short-lived however. The epidural started to leak after a couple of days and was removed. Pain management was now self-administered morphine.

The system is designed to prevent overdosing. I'm not convinced it really works. After a couple of days I began to see inanimate objects around the ward take on some sort of animate form. The first thing to metamorphose was the lamp on the nurses' desk, which turned into a penguin. A nurse was writing on a white board; her arm was above her head as she stretched to reach the top of the board. A stork. Annie would sit beside me as I pointed out the growing aviary to her. I felt completely sane and rational while this was going on. Although in truth, I could not have been entirely *compos mentis* because I was describing things to her as if she could see the same things as me. I guess it would have been worrying if she had.

My hallucinations were accompanied by clarity of sight and an increase in contrast between colours. I had never experience mind-altering drugs in the 60s but could now see how the senses could be enlightened by their use. The experience for me was entirely visual – I had hoped I would be able to write something like the *Sgt Pepper* album. But my song writing talent is severely lacking – even with the benefit of morphine.

My journey into the bizarre came to an end when I went to theatre for the ileostomy. It would be another chance for the epidural to manage the pain.

The food was so good – I just had to have it again

Late January 2006

I thought I had woken up in a scene from *CSI*; subdued blue lighting, torches, blue uniforms. I had no idea where I was. Annie was there and so was the Bag Lady. I couldn't speak and gestured for something to write with:

'Am I going to die?'
'I knew he was going to write that,' said Bag Lady.

I was reassured that I was not going to die – but I was in Intensive Care or more accurately the Critical Care Unit (CCU).

It was about 2.00 in the morning. Annie had been there since about midnight, in the relatives' room, surrounded by leaflets and posters offering advice on *'coping with bereavement'*. A good start.

I had faecal peritonitis – waste had leaked into the abdominal cavity. I couldn't understand how. I hadn't eaten for over a week and my system had been flushed through with *Kleen-Prep* (who thinks up these names?) Where was the waste coming from? It appears that waste can hide away in the nooks and crannies of our intestines for years. Short of a pressure washer up the back passage, we can never be completely clean inside.

CCU was an odd place. Nursing care is one-to-one (compared with around one nurse for every five or so beds on the ward). And the bed layout is more spacious allowing more privacy and more peace and quiet than on the ward. So it's definitely the place to be if you are ill. But that's the problem – if you are in CCU, you know you are ill.

Pain management was again an epidural. And again it leaked and so I was given morphine. In the next bay was a prisoner guarded by four police officers for a whole weekend. And me with my own stash of Class A drugs a few yards away.

This time the morphine did not have an hallucinogenic effect – it made me feel extremely unwell. I decided to come off it – and had withdrawal symptoms for over 24 hours. Not as bad as that scene from *Withnail and I*, but it made me realise what drug users go through when they try to kick the habit. An experience I would not wish to repeat. One of the doctors took pity on me and prescribed *Paracetamol IV* for pain relief. This is a very expensive form of the drug, administered intravenously and not to be given out readily. He had to 'borrow' it from one of the operating theatres. It was almost farcical – a doctor dealing black market drugs, while the police were next-door.

I found being in CCU difficult to begin with – I had expected to be going home about now and things were getting worse with no end in sight. I had a stoma bag, catheter and two tubes coming out of my stomach to drain the wounds. I was fed intravenously and the waste removed by a nurse. I had no control over what went into my body or what came out. This utter dependence on others was something I needed to come to terms with. When I was young my father had been dependant on my mother and me to feed and clean him and it was not something I had ever envisaged for myself.

In the end I just gave in to it. I managed to find an inner peace and adopted an almost beatific pose, smiling at all the doctors and nurses whenever they stopped by my bed. I can see why people become institutionalised; it's not so much giving up control that's scary – it's taking it back afterwards that becomes hard.

By this time the cancer had begun to decline in importance. Getting out of CCU became my priority. I'd spent a week on the ward before coming into CCU and it had taken its toll. My leg muscles had all but disappeared and breathing became an effort from lying horizontal for so long. I could sit in a chair for about an hour before needing to lie down again. I had been riding my bike on the morning that I came into hospital and I now began to wonder if I would ever ride it again. The lowest point came one night when one of the doctors making his rounds stopped for a chat. He told me my chances were 50:50 and perhaps I might want to think about '*alternatives*'. Alternative what? I'm not ashamed to admit I cried.

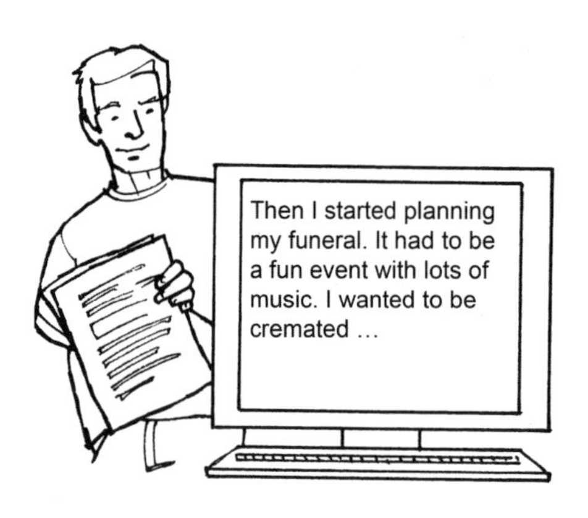

At first I felt utter despair. Then I started planning my funeral. It had to be a fun event with lots of music. I wanted to be cremated and when the coffin disappeared behind the curtain I wanted everyone to shout out '*encore*' and for it to reappear. The fact that Annie and I were planning a life together and that the band were enjoying such success only added to the poignancy of a life cut short. It seemed such a *rock 'n' roll* end.

I then realised that I had not told anyone of my wishes which meant I would not get the funeral I wanted. Not only that, I could not possibly die because the house was so untidy. Who would pay my credit card bills? Would Annie remember to put the rubbish out? Would she be able to manage the garage door? There were so many jobs that I had not got round to doing that she would not know about. A drainpipe had already fallen on her head.

I did everything I could that night to remain positive – I gave myself a good talking to and I prayed (and I'm not a religious man). I willed myself not to give in.

Up to this point I'd been sustained by intravenous (IV) fluids. They decided to try a liquid food (a misnomer if ever there was one) delivered through a tube up my nose. It was vanilla flavoured – although it was the smell and not the flavour I was aware of. They wanted to know if I had absorbed any of it or was it just passing through. So after a couple of hours one of the nurse stuck a pump down my throat, sucked out the contents of my stomach and went off to weigh it. She returned excitedly announcing that I'd absorbed 200gms. This was apparently a good thing. It meant that my body could take nutrients from food rather than IV fluids.

Then to Annie's utter horror and amazement she tipped the stuff that she'd just weighed back into the liquid food container – so I ended up having it again. Waste not, want not I guess.

About 10pm that night I had a craving for real food. The nurse went off to get me some cornflakes and milk. This is CCU room service. It seemed like the most wonderful thing I had ever tasted – I couldn't imagine the finest restaurant in the world serving anything better. Of course I threw it up, but that's not the point. It tasted good. I tried again next day at breakfast and it stayed down.

One of the things I dislike about being in hospital is the smell. The stoma bag smelt unpleasant when it was emptied and the smell coming from my drains was overpowering – like an abattoir (I used to live near one when I was young and you never forget the smell of dead meat). I talked to a doctor about it – he leaned over and whispered discreetly, while glancing at the person in the bed opposite – *'the thing you have to remember about being in hospital, is that the smell is not just you'.* While this was intended to reassure me, it completely changed my perception of the person opposite. I never looked on her in the same light again.

After ten days and a few helpings of hospital macaroni cheese and the chicken pasta dish that Annie bought in from *M&S*, they declared I should return to the ward. I viewed this news with mixed feelings. I would be returning to chaos. The staff in critical care were just wonderful. I knew I would simply not get that level of care and attention again. But it meant I was on the mend.

Postscript
I've just had letter from the Critical Care Unit inviting me to go back in a couple of weeks' time to give some feedback to the staff on my experience of being there. They say they never recognise the patients when they return, only the relatives. I wonder if they'll recognise my smell.

A quiet night in

Late January 2006

It's only when you're in hospital for any length of time that you really understand how it all works and what the staff, particularly the nurses have to deal with. And although the screens are meant to suggest privacy, you can still hear everything that goes on.

I arrived back in the ward from critical care to find two elderly gentlemen in the beds opposite. One immediately made me think – 'colonel'. He was in his late seventies, tall, slim, wore a cravat and one of those jumpers with elbow patches and shoulder patches. He had been a fighter pilot in the Second World War so perhaps 'wing commander' would have been more appropriate. I discovered that the nurses referred to him as 'the major'.

He was extremely fit – had a tumour removed by keyhole surgery and was home in five days (hmm). He was quite demanding, always calling for the nurses – at one time he asked a consultant (when accompanied by a large entourage) if he would take some money and fetch him some *Polo* mints from the hospital shop. The consultant just stared at him in utter disbelief – and ignored the request.

The other gentlemen was also demanding, but in a completely different way. He was striking because he was tall, upright, wore a long beard and spoke in a manner, which switched from quiet, sweet reasonableness to a terrifying roar. He was also striking because he scared the pants off me with his big stick. He was in his 90s; he was known as O.B. (as in *Obi-Wan Kenobi*).

They both arrived back in the ward from their respective operations in the evening. The colonel slept – his snoring amplified and given a more ominous tenor by the tubes in his nose and the oxygen mask covering his face. A nurse, making her twilight rounds, asked if I wanted a sleeping pill. I declined – apart from the rumble opposite, the ward was quiet for a change. A few nights before the fire alarm had gone off when an orderly left her bread too long in the toaster. And the previous night someone had raided the ward looking for drugs, hotly pursued by security staff. Somehow I imagined that this particular night held the promise of (relative) peace and quiet.

O.B. however did not sleep. Although weighed down by a catheter and drains he continually attempted to get out of bed. The nurses would catch sight of him and persuade him to get back in and go to sleep. But O.B. was not about to give up that easily and by about midnight he had made it. He ripped out the catheter and the various tubes and made off, unseen down the corridor. His escape route however was not hard to spot. A trail of urine, blood and other bodily fluids eventually gave him away.

It took three nurses to get him into bed. They were clearly exasperated but spoke to him with kindness, patience and good humour. He did not appreciate this and roared at them *'you can't talk to me like this, I used to be a school master'.* He let them subdue him and settled down. As soon as they had gone he was up again. This time he stuck the catheter and drains in the pockets of his dressing gown in what I imagine was an attempt to avoid leaving an obvious trail. He picked up his stick and wandered over to my bed. He waved it at my head demanding to know what I was doing in his house. Up to this point I had watched all this with an air of mild irritation at the disturbance to my sleep and amusement. Now I began to think – he might be 90 – but I would be in serious trouble if he decided to press for answers with his stick.

Another older man in the bed next to mine began to sing. He was asleep but singing. A clear, discernable if unrecognisable, tune. It made me wonder what our generation might sing in their sleep when they got to be elderly. What will turn out to be the sub-conscious soundtrack to our particular lives?

O.B. wandered over to the colonel's bed and demanded to know why he was also in his house. At this point the colonel woke up and stared shouting:

'Nurse – I want my teeth.'
'You won't be needing them for a while dear, you can't eat anything.'

A passing nurse delivered this line in such a matter of fact way — as if it was something she did on a regular basis.

At this point I regretted not taking up the offer of a sleeping pill. Nurses continued to put O.B. to bed and he continued to thwart them. At some point they must have tucked the sheets in tight because he eventually gave up. But the promise of a quiet night had all but gone.

Before too long the noise level in the ward gradually increased. The day shift began to wander in ready for handover from the night shift. A distant rumble signalled the arrival of the tea trolley and doctors and other members of the various consultants' teams were gathering their notes, checking for any problems noted by the night shift, in anticipation of 'the rounds'. The noise level would reach a climax before falling away as the caravan moved on. This particular morning, having had my breakfast, I put on the headphones from the radio in order to drown out the background noise, gazed out of the window and dropped off to sleep.

Over the next few days and nights O.B.'s wanderlust only increased. Sometimes he would wander the ward searching for his dog. But at other times he would be found, clearly troubled, in the toilet. The nurses explained countless times that he did not need to go to the loo because he had a catheter. This did not satisfy O.B. He was in pain and the catheter was not working. Then, one evening, behind the screens, a nurse found the problem: *'You've got a knot in your catheter'.*

Just how this occurred was the subject of much speculation — but never satisfactorily explained.

Time to go home

Early February 2006

From the time I arrived back on the ward I campaigned to go home. I would tell anyone who would listen – passing doctors, nurses, visitors – that I needed an end date for my stay. Of course it's not as simple as that. For a start, I had been weakened by my stay in hospital. I still had a catheter and drains attached. And I could walk no further than the end of the bed – and only then with the physiotherapist to help me. The combination of so little exercise and the high fat, high protein, no fibre diet meant that what weight I had gained had accumulated around the middle and I now looked like a straw stuck through a ping-pong ball.

The days were starting to get me down. I didn't have the energy to read and daytime television was simply dire. I was fortunate to have a bed by a window and could watch the grey skies keep their monotonous monochrome hue. Whatever happened to bright, sunny, crisp winter mornings? (I realise that being a patient means being patient.)

A typical day would begin at 6.00am with blood pressure and temperature readings. Drugs would be administered. The subdued night-time lighting would abruptly end with the switching on of the overhead fluorescents. *Wakey, wakey, rise and shine*. I would doze intermittently until the arrival of the tea trolley signalled the proper start to the hospital day.

I had developed a taste for cornflakes and cold milk. No idea why – it's not something I ever have at home. I always awoke hungry and eager for the arrival of the breakfast trolley around 8.00am. About 9.00am the doctors would do their rounds.

Sometimes this would be a low-key affair, perhaps involving just a couple of people. The consultants would usually come round twice a week bringing with them a crowd of hangers on. I always found this a fascinating process. The consultant would first address me then the crowd, switching code between technical and non-technical language. I was able to keep up to some extent with the jargon. The medical profession has made a real attempt to communicate with patients and now explains things more fully. Just how much we actually take in is arguable; as patients we're expected to do our bit. We have to do our homework, usually via the Internet, to ensure a proper two-way conversation.

Next on the agenda was bath-time — usually around 10.00. With luck this could easily last until 11.00. On my first morning back in the ward a nurse asked what arrangements I had made for washing while I'd been in critical care. The purpose of this question was to find out if I could get myself to the bathroom or whether I'd need a bed bath. From the busy nurses' point of view a visit to the bathroom gave them time to make the beds. I replied that I had been bathed in asses' milk by handmaidens: *'You're not in ****** critical care now, you'll make do with me and a rub down with a flannel'.*

A bed bath is a humiliation. Although the nurses are kind and do it with patience and good humour there is no getting round the loss of dignity. The humiliation was compounded in my case when I had to ask them to empty my bag. I could wait up to an hour if they were especially busy. One particular nurse always delayed this task — *'I'll do it later - can't face it first thing - puts me off my breakfast'.* Hmm. Me too.

I gradually learned to sit on the side of the bed and wash myself. Once clean and with a freshly made bed, I would sit in the chair until lunchtime.

Lunch arrived at 12.00 and was finished by about ten past. Washing, sitting in a chair for an hour and eating was exhausting at first and I was relieved to get back into bed. It was not difficult to doze off until visiting time at 3.00pm.

A physiotherapist would usually come round in the afternoon and coax me out of bed. I was always reluctant, but knew I had to do it if I were to be allowed home. At first I had a walking frame for support and then a walking stick (watch out O.B., my turn now). I stooped as I walked, my chest fighting for breath. I felt ancient. Progress was slow, but progress was made. One day Annie arrived to see me walk from one side of the ward to the other – about 30 feet, but it could have been 30 miles as far as I was concerned.

Visiting time ended at 5.00pm in time for supper. Another doze until visitors were allowed back in at 7.00pm. As my appetite improved, Annie would bring in treats; warm roast chicken or sausage sandwiches in fresh white crusty bread, *Ben & Jerry's* chocolate ice cream, a bag of crisps and a tin of peaches and pears. This was the life.

All too quickly it was over – the bell sounded at 8.00, a signal that it was time for her to go. Left alone, the atmosphere, like the patients, quickly became subdued. Some watched television, but others, like me, just lay there waiting for tomorrow.

By about the third week I was starting to get frustrated; the drains could not come out because they were still discharging stuff that should not be in my body. I hated them. Apart from the smell, they were heavy when full and pulled on my skin when I moved. To walk I had to gather them up, one in either hand, with the catheter slung over the front of the walking frame. The eventual removal of the catheter (which did not hurt, but felt really weird) meant one less thing to worry about. This freed me up to walk to the bathroom.

Going to the bathroom myself was another important step on the road to recovery. I no longer had to wait for someone to take a full bottle away and bring a new one. The fact that I could manage to get to the bathroom prompted a nurse to ask one morning if I would like to try having a shower. This was a big deal. I had not had a shower (or a proper hair wash) for over three weeks. I had to think about it. Once I'd agreed I became really excited, even though I had to wait for two hours for a nurse to be free to carry my wash things (two drains was enough for me to manage). It completely altered my day – my mood changed out of all proportion of the event – I was only having a shower. It's what people do every day.

It had to be planned carefully. The drains were emptied so that I would not have to deal with the weight. But they were long – the tubes ran from my stomach down to the floor. I thought about taping them to my legs so I would not have to hold on to them while in the shower. The nurses were not happy about this, thinking that the tape would lose its grip when wet. One suddenly had a brainwave and rushed off. She came back with two pairs of surgical knickers. I couldn't work out what she had in mind other than it was bound to be humiliating.

She took one pair, twisted them into a figure of eight and folded them over so that they now had one opening instead of two. She slipped them over my left leg stopping just above the knee. It looked just like a giant garter. She then coiled up the tubes and tucked them in. Satisfied, she did the same with the right leg. I looked ridiculous. You have to bear in mind I'm wearing a hospital gown (the type that opens at the back) – and being taller than average, it looks not unlike a mini-dress popular among Modish women in the 1960s. But I'm no Mary Quant and I was past caring – I just wanted that shower.

Undressing in the bathroom was a shock. I had not seen myself naked for weeks. I had lost so much weight Evelyn Glennie would get a decent tune out of my ribs. My beard had grown thick. And I smelled. It was an effort to stand upright, the combination of dressings, drains and the bag pulling the skin tight, but the water felt good running down my hair and back. I was almost overcome at the achievement.

I lay down on the bed when I returned and waited for the wet dressings to be changed. And there I stayed for the rest of the day. My first proper attempt at cleanliness had been exhausting. My stomach muscles ached the next day from being stretched beyond their normal range of movement.

On my 26th day in hospital the consultant agreed that I could go home in the next few days. Suddenly everything changed. The drains were removed (it didn't hurt – but removing the stitches that held them in place did), the IV antibiotics were stopped along with other medication. No more washes at the bedside; I was expected to use the bathroom. Two physios came and took me by wheelchair to a stairwell. I was invited to climb up and down – which I managed to do after a fashion. They ticked the boxes and left.

Like I said before, it's not so much giving up control that's daunting – it's taking it back afterwards that becomes hard. Because when control is given back it all happens very quickly.

There was one last thing to deal with. The bag. I would not be allowed home unless the Bag Lady was satisfied I could change the bag and clean my stoma. No matter what the consultant said, she would have the last word.

Up to this point I had avoided having anything to do with it. Nurses emptied it when they had time, but now I had to take responsibility. I talked to the Bag Lady and agreed a strategy – a two-day course of action. On day one I would practise emptying it and day two I would, under her supervision, change it. Emptying it was OK. I was glad not having to rely on others. I quickly learned how to squat on the loo seat to avoid getting splashed. Changing it was a different matter. I had not even looked at the stoma.

The Bag Lady was a brilliant tutor. She understood my reluctance and took me through the process with great patience. I had to confront it to clean it. It looked so weird. It could move in an out, seemingly under its own volition. My main concern was what to do if it leaked into the dressing. It had leaked on a number of occasions, usually at night when I was asleep. My wound was already infected as a result. I'm suddenly responsible for my own well-being, which is scary having been dependent on others for so long. She reassured me that a district nurse would call daily to change the dressings and she would visit me at home in a week's time.

I was presented with a hand bag – in a rather fetching shade of pale blue – containing all the paraphernalia for changing the stoma bag, including spare bags, wipes and scissors for cutting a hole in the bag to fit my individual stoma. It felt like some sort of reward or passing out prize. I would be free to go home before lunch on Thursday February 9th. I had spent 29 days in hospital including ten in critical care.

On my last morning the bag leaked as I waited for the dressings to be changed. As the nurse was cleaning up, she looked at my stoma:

'Oh this is really good, this is beautiful'.

I looked her full in the face. She returned my stare – thought for a minute and then said:

'I suppose my idea of beauty is different from yours?' I have this thing, which looks a bit like a tongue with a hole in it sticking out of my belly, and she's talking aesthetics.

Being here has been an education. I've learned such a lot – about myself as much as how the NHS works. No matter how bad I've felt – both physically and emotionally – there are people much worse off than me. I wake up each day grateful and pleased to still be here. Compared with some I've got off lightly.

Doctors and nurses work incredibly hard and have a lot to deal with. We expect them to know all the answers. But they can't – because we can't always articulate accurately enough how we're feeling or what is happening to us.

In spite of the fact that illness is a 24/7 activity, the NHS does not operate on a 24/7 basis. It does not pay to be admitted on a Friday. X-Rays have priority but it'll be Monday before other tests can be done – unless they can find someone to work overtime.

To be fair, the NHS is doing its bit. In what I can only assume is an attempt to solve its financial crisis, hospitals are now employing maggots as part of a *'wound management system'* (Maggot Debridement Therapy). This is true. Apparently the little bugs have been especially trained to nibble away at infected (dark) skin tissue and thereby expose the good (red) skin tissue underneath. I'm told they are very effective.

They're distinguishable from their everyday detritus-eating cousins because they have a red cross on their back. This is the NHS's only concession to a uniform. The maggots' trade union, **MITES** (**M**iniature **I**nsectivorous bio**ThE**rapeutic **S**taff, also representing leeches and other members of the biotherapeutic community) had hoped for miniature stethoscopes to sling round their shoulders, but funding would not stretch this far – even though it's a very, very short distance.

Stair-lift to heaven

Early February 2006

Coming home was an emotional experience. Annie had prepared a warm welcome, flowers, cards from well-wishers and a tub of ice-cream.

She'd made up a bed downstairs because I was not confident I could manage the stairs, in spite of my successful attempt in hospital. It's a lot different when there's a big, strong physio waiting at the bottom to catch you if you fall.

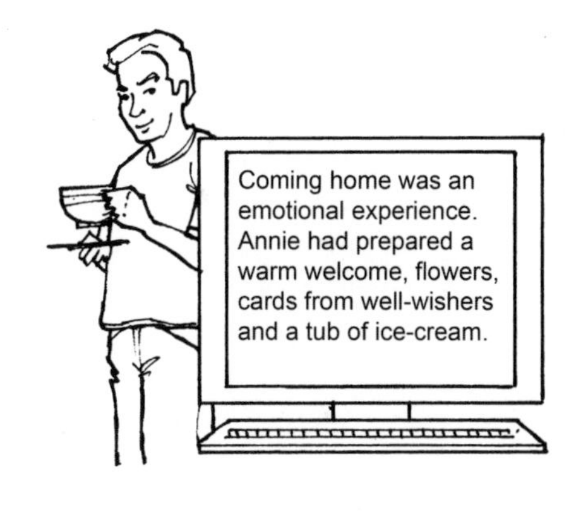

Four weeks was not the longest I'd been away from home, but there were times when I did wonder if I'd see it again. I sat looking out at the garden just taking it all in.

I cried many times over the first weekend – probably from the stress of coming out and the sheer joy and relief at being home. Up to that point my entire world had been limited to a bed and a chair. Now I had rooms to sit in as well as a selection of beds and chairs. I was spoilt for choice.

Someone said that they admired my courage for the way I had dealt with this. It has nothing to do with courage. Courage or bravery has an element of choice about it – we can *choose* whether or not to go into the burning building. I, like many others, have no choice. We just have to get on with it. The Bag Lady has around five hundred patients on her books; these are people living with the consequences of a colostomy or an ileostomy. The youngest (at the time we talked) was six weeks old. If medals for courage are to be handed out, then surely they go to all those who watch and wait. I would guess they feel helpless because they cannot change the course of the disease – only deal with its fallout.

The hero of my story is Annie. This has been as much a shock for her as it has been for me. It's changed her life as much as mine. I've had all the attention, with plenty of people to care and look after me. But she's had to go home alone each night. When I was in critical care she was told my chances were 50:50 before I was. So to come back day after day, not knowing what to expect, takes real courage.

That night I stood at the bottom of the stairs, getting the measure of it. Oh for a lift to whizz me up and down. In the end I decided to give it a go. I would only have to do this twice a day – once going up and once coming down. Walking stick in my right hand, banister rail in my left, I gingerly made my way up. I felt an immense sense of satisfaction at the top. When times are bad there is no place like your own bed. Heaven.

Nurse Gladys Emmanuel

Mid February 2006

I have to confess that, at the moment, life with a bag is a bit of a drag. I still haven't properly bonded with it. It took me more than three weeks before I could even look at it (a mix of squeamishness and denial I guess). The first time I changed one on my own, I forgot to do up the *Velcro* flap at the bottom (through which it empties) – remembered just in time to stop a nasty mess from running down my leg.

I have to empty it about three times during the night and around half a dozen times during the day. The small colon sure is a busy old thing. I change the bag every other day.

The other complication is that I still have two open wounds in my abdomen and the dressings overlap with where the sticky backing of the bag needs to be. If I don't attach it properly the bag will leak – as happened yesterday morning. The mess I can cope with – the worry is that it leaks into one of the wounds. The main wound from the first operation has still not healed – in fact it has an infection – the result of which is what the district nurse calls 'a malodorous discharge'. The dressing leaks down my legs which is just plain unpleasant.

I'm managing to walk around the house without the stick. I can now get up off the sofa without someone helping me, although I still make a noise. (A sign of ageing is when you can't get up from a low chair without grunting, wheezing, sighing ... or generally making a song and dance about it.)

The mornings are particularly good for me. The district nurse comes around midday to change the dressings and after that I'm done for. There's a lot of pushing and prodding to get rid of the malodorous discharge and afterwards I just want to go to bed with a couple of painkillers. It's as if my internal organs have been rearranged from the outside.

When I was told that a district nurse would come out to change the dressings, my immediate thought was of Nurse Gladys Emmanuel (*Open All Hours*) – buxom female, hair in a bun and driving a Morris Minor or riding a bike with a basket on the front. I soon dismissed that as a stereotype at least 30 years old. I was still not prepared however for the district nurse who did turn up – more Bob Marley than Gladys Emmanuel. About 90% of the nurses in the hospital appeared to be female, so I just assumed that the district nurse would be female. But I shouldn't really have been surprised, should I?

In the event I would see about six different district nurses (the other five were female), but he would be my main carer. He was kind, caring and I am grateful to him because he made a significant difference to my recovery.

Mr Creosote

Early March 2006

It's been three days since I've had a 'malodorous discharge' from the wound. So I think things are looking up. I'm feeling better and starting to get a bit more adventurous.

I woke up on Sunday to find that the bag had leaked in the night. It had made more of a mess than usual and I had to take the dressings off. Fortunately the wound was clean but that was about all. The only way I could clean up was to sit in the bath. So, circumstances forced the next big test. The district nurse was due that morning to change the dressings, so I knew if I got stuck Annie would have help in getting me out. It was not a luxurious soak, I couldn't risk getting water in the wound – but enough to reacquaint my undercarriage with soap and water. Bliss. As it turns out I couldn't get out without help, but it's a start.

I've started playing the guitar and singing again. This leads to an unexpected discovery – my stoma has rhythm. Singing moves the diaphragm, which moves the stomach, which moves the small colon ... and the stoma kicks into action. This is going to be something to see on stage.

I'm starting to put on weight. I don't know how much I weighed when I came out of hospital, I would guess less than 11st. I'm 11st 4lb at the moment. It's still accumulating around my middle. Instead of the 'straw through a ping-pong ball' I now look like a straw through a tennis ball. Annie bought me some new tracksuit bottoms – she had to get a size 42" waist, because a 36" waist was too tight – I kid you not. This on someone 6'2" and just over 11st. It must be the bag and dressings that are fat. Or I'm turning into Mr Creosote *('just another wafer thin mint?')*.

The good, the bad and the ugli (fruit)

Early March 2006

There is definitely a good time and a bad time to change the stoma bag. The best time I find is late morning. I usually do it somewhere quiet where I can lay out all the necessary bits and pieces – clean bag, adhesive remover, odour-proof disposal bag for the mucky bits, clean wipes, a bowl of warm water and a cup of tea. I take my time as I learn to bond with my stoma. We are learning much about each other. We may not stay together, but we'll part with no regrets.

The worst time is at 3.30 in the morning when the bag has sprung a leak. It's happened enough times now that I've got it off to a fine art – perched on the loo-seat half asleep, trying to remember the nappy-changing mantra (*wipe once, wipe away*) – and failing to stop the stuff going down my legs, because I had supper later than usual and the stoma is active.

A stoma is a bit like a volcano. It lies dormant for ages then erupts – not in a spectacular explosive Krakatoa fashion, but more like the volcanoes of Hawaii. And like a volcano – eruptions from the stoma are extremely hard to predict. In fact the only real way of telling what's going on is when the old bag is off and Mauna Loa is still chucking it out. As it was this morning.

Three hands would be useful at this stage. One to stem the flow while the other two manipulate the new bag into place. Perhaps if there's no cure for bowel cancer, we'll need to evolve that third hand.

I think I've discovered a flaw in the bag design. The bag is roughly eight inches long, flesh-coloured (although if you saw anyone with flesh that colour you might fear for their health – or suggest they have words with their make-up adviser) with an opening at the bottom, secured by a *Velcro* flap. What trust we place in hooks and loops.

On the back at the top is a round sticky pad about three inches in diameter with a hole cut in it for the stoma to poke through. On the front is a charcoal filter to cut down on bad smells.

The bag works fine when I'm upright – sitting or walking about – gravity delivers the contents to where it should be. But when I'm horizontal I lose that benefit. The stuff piles upwards instead, eventually blocking the charcoal filter and the bag fills with gas. It can't get out through the flap at the bottom, so it seeps out underneath the sticky pad, usually into the dressing, which is about an inch away.

I've been having really bad stomach pains recently – coinciding with the start of a powerful new antibiotic to deal with the wound infection. The antibiotic was stopped but the pain persisted. As a result I've lost my appetite, which is cause for concern. Medical opinion was divided for about a week (the most popular theory being that antibiotics take ages to leave the system) but the latest thinking is that perhaps the high fat diet has caused problems for the gall bladder. So I have a week's trial of no cheese or milk (which I've been consuming in vast quantities) to see if that makes a difference.

The novelty of the Homer Simpson diet (high fat, high protein, no fibre) is starting to wear off. I'm bored with burgers. I keep fantasizing about apples. When all this is over the first thing I'm going to eat is an apple. I'm allowed to eat root vegetables so, in a bid to eat something fresh, I had a raw carrot and celeriac salad. Big mistake. It came out pretty much as it went in – completely undigested. When mixed with the other contents of the bag it achieved a consistency that would enable it to be used successfully to renovate the walls of a medieval building.

Pushing the boundaries of my diet has paid off and I've discovered I can eat mango. Oh what joy this brings. Mango is wonderful. So I can now increase my intake of fruit to include raspberries (remembering to chew the pips) blueberries and mango. Bliss.

I don't like Mondays (tell me why)

Mid March 2006

Sundays are turning out to be my favourite day of the week. Weekdays begin far too early and there's too much frantic activity (though not from me). Saturdays begin perhaps an hour or so later, and although the pace is not so fast, there's shopping, washing, etc. to catch up on. But Sundays have a pace and rhythm all their own.

Sundays begin with tea in bed. This is a big change. When I had my dog I was up and out by about 7.30 every day. But tea in bed is a real treat and a very civilised way of greeting the day. I wonder if this will continue once I'm 'back to normal'?

While Annie makes breakfast (mango, blueberries, raspberries, strawberries, melon and yogurt – mmm) I have a bath. Still not yet the lingering soak, but enough to give some semblance of normality. Although I can get into the bath myself, I can't yet get out without help – perhaps the next indicator of progress is when I can achieve this.

I change the bag and by the time we've had breakfast the district nurse is here to change the dressings. So, by about half past ten I'm fed, clean and ready for what else the day has to offer. Lunch usually.

When I was having difficulty eating a few weeks ago, the Bag Lady suggested roast dinners. What a revelation. So Sunday lunch now consists of roasted root vegetables (potatoes, sweet potatoes, swede, parsnips and carrots) with gravy and a portion of happy chicken, happy cow, happy pig or happy lamb.

Lunch is usually followed by a walk or visitors. Late afternoon Annie starts marking homework and lesson-planning. Such is a schoolteacher's lot. And I have a nap. Can't complain really. It's a good life.

But I don't like Mondays. Annie's up at 6.30 and out of the door by 8.00. I get up before she goes, we have breakfast together, then the front door closes and it's quiet. Now what? I've got to that stage where I'm feeling so much better and want to do things but don't have the energy. The band came round on Saturday morning – and although I only sang a few songs, I suffered for it in the afternoon. Not just exhaustion – the stomach muscles still haven't fully healed up yet from surgery. I feel like I've done 100 press-ups.

The nurse has just been round to change the dressings. He's given me the news I've long been dreading – he's not coming tomorrow. My malodorous discharge is (a) no longer malodorous and (b) not discharging. He'll only come once a week from now on. I am officially on the mend.

The wrong trousers

Late March 2006

I've got into the habit of weighing myself on Sunday mornings before I have a bath. We have these new super-duper scales which not only indicate your weight but also body fat, % muscle content and % water content as well as life expectancy, sexual orientation, political allegiance and who's likely to get evicted from the Big Brother house.

This Sunday I weighed in at 12st 4lb – a gain of over 4lb on the week. I think most of this can be attributed to a beef stew with dumplings and Rocky Road pudding the previous day; I'll wait for confirmation next Sunday.

This gain in weight, while indicating a return to health has its drawbacks. As I've mentioned before, most of the additional weight is accumulating around the middle. Lack of exercise is preventing its redistribution to more needy parts of my anatomy. The problem is clothes – specifically trousers.

Those who've been to visit may have noticed that I tend to appear in loose fitting tracksuits (a far cry from my usual sartorial elegance). It's a new style – *post-op grunge*. Annie's eldest, Chris and his girlfriend Emma, have invited us out to dinner to celebrate Mother's Day. I can hardly wear my usual attire. So getting trousers to fit (over the bag as well) will be a challenge.

Going out to dinner will also be a challenge. The first time I went out in the car the motion caused the dressings to leak and the seatbelt is tight across the bag. I've just been reading about a man whose bag burst while he was driving his car. At least it's a better excuse for erratic driving than using a mobile.

When you're coping with cancer there's a lot of emphasis on pain management, but nothing on pants management. I find the emotional aspects of living with the disease harder than some of the physical aspects. I can accept pain because it's something I expected to happen. It goes with the territory and the drugs control it (eventually). But I get upset when the bag leaks and I mess my pants. I didn't think it was going to be like this. They don't prepare you for these aspects of bag-life.

The other thing they don't prepare you for is the smell, although perhaps I should have guessed. My stoma care bag contains amongst other things a discreet little spray called 'pouch deodorant'. Sounds innocuous but it's powerful stuff. And it needs to be.

So I'm apprehensive about being out in public. I get very self-conscious. First thing I always do is check the loos. Is there room to empty/change the bag? Will I leave a bad smell? Will I mess my pants? Will I get funny looks walking around with an attention-grabbing pale blue handbag?

But it's progress. And I no longer have dressings on the wound. So I can shower. Another step forward. The next hurdle will be the liver surgery.

Now I think about it, the next hurdle will not be liver surgery. The band have a gig on Good Friday. I've agreed to do a few songs. That's my next challenge. My stoma and I are really looking forward to it.

Good to hear from you and a blog is certainly is the best way to communicate/share with everyone. I am very impressed with your writing skills – your ability to express the reality (pain, humour, acceptance, and strength) of life in IC.

Dave
28th March 2006

Just an ordinary day

April 1st 2006

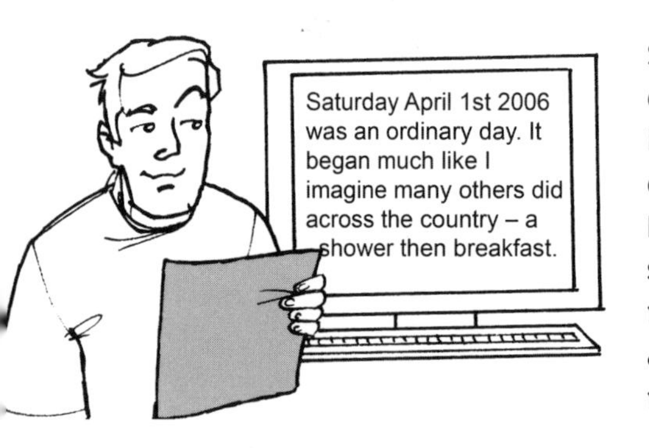

Saturday April 1st 2006 was an ordinary day. It began much like I imagine many others did across the country – a shower then breakfast. Later that morning I drove to the shops, bought half a dozen items and returned in time for lunch. In the afternoon, while Annie pruned the roses, I put up a shelf in the garage.

We shared a bottle of wine with our supper, read, watched a bit of television then went to bed. I fell asleep lying on my side. Like I said, just an ordinary day.

Except this time last week I couldn't drive the car, go shopping, drill holes in the garage wall or sleep on my side.

It's been three months since I've visited a supermarket. It's a challenge at first – some of the things I wanted are on the bottom shelf and I struggle to reach them. Then the bag needs emptying. No panic. I choose a disabled loo to give myself bit more space to sort myself out. All well and good until I discover that the toilet roll is jammed up inside the dispenser. I manage to shove my hand up inside and pull on the tissue. It unwinds then breaks. So I shove my hand up again, grab some tissue, pull it and it breaks again. All the while I'm having to keep the bag pointed into the pan to stop the contents escaping elsewhere.

It makes me think about disabled people. I'm able-bodied, but how would someone less mobile than me manage in this situation? Perhaps they're used to it. It's all new to me so I'm seeing what others have to deal with for the first time.

The other thing that strikes me is just how rude and ill-mannered people are. Were they always like that or am I seeing this for the first time as well?

I realise that I too have become rude and impatient. I was not at all like this in hospital. I was a model patient – calm and serene. As I write this, Annie comes to see what I'm up to. I tell her that I'm writing about my ill-temper – she offers to confirm it for anyone who can't believe it.

In the end I put this change down to frustration. My body has not caught up with my brain. I feel fine – in my head I am back to normal and can now get on and do things. But I can't pick up something from the bottom shelf of a supermarket. When I get back from the shops I have to lie down for half an hour. And so I now have a new worry – people who see me out and about will think I'm skiving off work. Perhaps I could wear a sign that indicates my progress – 'almost but not quite recovered – honest'.

But thinking about it, this is a good problem to have. And so April 1st was not an ordinary day after all. It was an extraordinary day.

What not to wear

April 2nd 2006

Having worked in television and performed in a band, I know just how important rehearsals are. Things cannot be left to the last minute. So I considered it necessary to do a full dress rehearsal – or rather full trouser rehearsal – before my first attempt at going out to dinner.

I had a number of options – jeans, cargoes, smart casual, formal and my ace in the hole – Rohan Uplanders with elasticated waistband.

I laid the various trousers out on the bed and inspected them. I wondered what Trinny and Susannah would say. Perhaps I could be their biggest challenge (or nightmare) – 'you'll never get shoes to match *that* bag'.

Jeans were the first to go – this was really wishful thinking on my part. Gradually the others were whittled away. Some even made it to the Oxfam bag. In some cases the waistband was too low and cut right across the bag. Others were just too tight. Although I was over a stone lighter than I had been before the operation, my waist was bigger.

Finally it was just the Rohans that were left. If they're good enough for scrambling round the French Alps and then a French restaurant they'll be good enough for the local carvery. I almost didn't bother to try them, such was my confidence. When they wouldn't do up I assumed Annie was holding them at the back as some sort of joke. But no.

I lay down on the bed and attempted to wriggle into them like a teenager who'd soaked their Levis in the bath to get a really tight fit. The waistband was high enough to clear the bag. Eventually I got the button done up. Only trouble now was that I could not get up off the bed. Nor could I bend down to put my shoes on. My range of movement in the vertical plane was limited to between 12 and 2 o'clock. And I had thought it was all going to be a piece of cake. That was obviously the problem – cake. And all the other things I'd eaten.

I can't work out if I've got fatter in real terms or if my stomach is still swollen from the effects of surgery. Or perhaps the muscles that were severed simply haven't healed yet and I wonder if the happy, smiling people in the '*living with an ileostomy*' brochure had to buy new trousers.

After helping me off the bed and on with my shoes, Annie took me for a drive. This was a proper rehearsal after all. I was folded into the car and strapped in. I just sat there staring straight ahead, unable to move one way or another. Although I needed help getting in and out, walking around was not too difficult – sitting was the problem (and so would eating be later on – which was the whole point of the exercise).

I then began to feel that familiar warm, damp sensation. We got home in time; the leak was in its infancy. So, back to the 42" waist tracksuit and post-op grunge. I'm going to have to go on a diet. Sometime.

Wow Ian – I loved this latest one!! You are amazing – you have stayed strong in dire circumstances and still seen the ridiculous humour and humanity in it all … almost made me feel nostalgic for nursing … I used to enjoy it so much … you really made it all come alive! I see the movie using the 'Peep Show' format … lots of inner thinking going on for the characters … and you played by Donald Sutherland!! Will be good when you catch up as I will then know what is going on NOW! Call anytime you fancy a chat … am back at work next week … six weeks of rest and relaxation (ho hum – NOT!!) it will be truly weird!! Take care of you … big hugs as always.

Nicola
5th April 2006

Here we go again

April 9th 2006

Every year around Easter time one of Mother Nature's most enduring spectacles takes place. It is as timeless and predictable as the black stork crossing the Bosphorus or the snow goose on its way north for the summer.

In the UK, scores of households eagerly await the emergence from hibernation of the *Power Tool*. In sheds, garages and under-stairs cupboards, electric drills, jigsaws and sanders awake from months of dormancy. The patient observer might even catch sight of the *lesser-spotted router* (so named because it is not seen that often, belonging to the genus *impulse-buy* — being distantly related to the electric sandwich-maker, corn-on-the cob skewers and the fondue set).

The reason for the excitement is the annual springtime ritual of DIY. Do-it-Yourself — or Bodge-it-Yourself as it is known in the trade — is the process whereby perfectly good houses are knocked about — walls taken out, walls put in, last year's bathroom replaced by this year's — in order to empty the shelves of DIY superstores.

This need — and it is a need — is deep-seated within the human psyche. It is no coincidence that many power tools look like weapons — indeed in the wrong hands they can become weapons of mass destruction. We wear them slung round our waists in tool holsters. The more reckless of the breed — the cowboy builder — has set him/herself free from the umbilical of the power lead and gone cordless. They might wear a drill on one side, a nail gun on the other with a mobile phone cunningly hidden behind their back in case of trouble. It seems that as we've become more civilised, the need to destroy people has been replaced by the need to destroy houses.

Annie and I are not immune from this need. We too have poured excitedly over paint cards, re-charged the screwdriver batteries and sharpened our saws as we 're-model' the house (as our American friends would say). We're painting, decorating, moving things around and generally having a good time. I say we — Annie is doing most of the hard labour — but I supervise, pointing out helpfully when she's missed a bit of paint or splashed a bit on the floor. It seems to work, because she gets on very quietly while I'm making the tea or strolling round the garden.

The reason for doing this now is two-fold. We were hoping to sell both our houses and buy a new one. Annie arranged the sale of hers, but the vendor of the house we agreed to buy sold to someone else (for more money) while I was in hospital. Another lesser-known side-effect of cancer – *gazumping*. We've looked around, but can't find anything we like that we can afford: we don't want to commit ourselves to a more expensive house while we live with all this uncertainty. So Plan B is to live in my house while we take stock and make plans. And we're re-modelling to make it *our* house instead of mine.

The other reason for doing it now is that I'm not that far away from liver surgery. And I need to do things while I'm able to, and to keep my mind off going back into hospital. And that process starts today with a PET (Positron Emission Tomography) scan. First I get to lie in a darkened room while radioactive glucose is injected into my body (it only has a half life of 2.5 hours so it's no big deal). The major side effect is boredom. I'm not allowed to move or read. Then a trip to the loo and into the machine.

The PET scan produces a 3D image of the cancer cells in the liver. So it will show the size, distribution and number of cells to be dealt with. I get the results on the 22nd when I meet with the consultant to plan the next stage. So – here we go again.

Good Friday – bad Friday

April 16th 2006

Most people I've come across with a life-threatening illness always advocate making the most of life; *'you never know what's round the corner'*. When they say things like this they tend to think at the macro level – they mean not putting off the grand plans, the things they've always wanted to do but never found the time, money or perhaps even courage. But the fickleness of life can also operate at the micro level. Things can be all right one day and not the next.

I've felt great the past two weeks. Driving has given me some independence and tinkering with the house has continued to reassure me that I'm on the mend. There's a four cubic yard builders' skip in the drive and I'm filling it with rubbish — old bits of wood that I saved for some purpose so long ago that I've quite forgotten what it was, half empty tins of dried-up paint and the stuff which just seems to accumulate over time as if by itself. Clearing out is therapeutic in itself, but I get an added pleasure from the fact that I can now manage to do this.

On Thursday 13th Annie and I went to visit the Critical Care Unit at the hospital. We'd been invited as part of programme of feeding back to staff and a chance to understand what, for many, is an extremely traumatic process. It was a very strange experience — for a start I had no idea where in the hospital the unit was — I'd been unconscious when I arrived. Secondly, it looked so bright and airy — quite unlike my recollection, which was of a blue ambience. We walked around the unit and as predicted, the nurses did not recognise me until they realised who Annie was. Then they commented how fit and well I looked.

That evening I went to a rehearsal at Neil's house (Neil being the mandolin player in *Fat Freddy's Cat*). The band has a gig booked for Good Friday and I have agreed to join them for a couple of songs. The rehearsal gave me sufficient confidence to do more than just a couple of songs. I mentioned that I'd like to come on at the end of the evening so that I could turn up at the last minute. This was not so that I could make a grand entrance (note to self: cancel request for them to play *Fanfare for the Common Man* as I make my way to the stage), but so I would not have to make a grand exit.

I explained how the stoma seems to pump (i.e. fill the bag) when I'm singing and that I did not want this to happen on stage in case of accidents. (Also — my ego is too big to share the stage with a star-struck stoma.) If I timed my meals right, it should be empty by the time I planned to turn up. We then talked about what I'd been doing to the house recently and my general level of fitness. This prompted the following interchange between Neil and myself:

Neil: *'So how are you feeling in yourself?'*
Me: *'I filled a skip this morning.'*

Neil looks at me quizzically.

Me: *'OK – so it was only one brick at a time, but I still managed to fill it.'*
Neil: *'Oh – I thought you meant from your bag.'*

On the Friday morning I put a few odds and ends of wood into the skip and then had breakfast. About ten minutes later I began to feel ill with severe stomach pains. I eventually went to bed. I'd had a similar pain about four weeks ago and could get no definitive diagnosis. It could be an adverse reaction to antibiotics (unlikely now), an ulcer, irritation of the gall bladder, something to do with the wound infection (again unlikely now), a stomach bug or something completely unknown. A doctor at the hospital said he simply could not say.

It feels like being punched in the stomach. Eating and drinking make it worse as does lying on my side. Someone said that this, together with the messiness of leaking bags, should give me some idea what women go through every month. Fair enough, but this is not what I expected to happen to me now – at 58.

As the day wore on I began to wonder if I would make it to the gig. I kept thinking of the song *'what a difference a day makes, 24 little hours'*. It just doesn't seem possible to be feeling so good one day and so bad the next. Last time this happened the pain would usually pass in about six hours or so, but it took over a week to disappear altogether.

I take some anti-acid pills in case it is the gall bladder secreting excess acid to counter the excess fat in my diet. No effect. I also take painkillers. No effect. By late afternoon I manage some dry toast and green tea.

I eventually get up about 7.30. I need to be at the gig by 10.00. I know I have a problem because the stoma has slowed down. Breakfast (fruit and yoghurt) usually puts in an appearance within two to three hours. Things only start to get moving around 8.00pm, a good five hours later than normal. I start to get anxious about the gig; will I have the energy? And more to the point – will the bag behave?

I shower then lie on the bed summoning up the energy to do this. I want so much to play and I know people will be expecting me to put in an appearance. I don't want to let them down. I learnt early on that playing gigs is about the audience, not the band. Too many bands are self-indulgent, playing just what they want to play without a thought for those who've made the effort to come and see them. We can be self-indulgent too – but we make sure we entertain people at the same time.

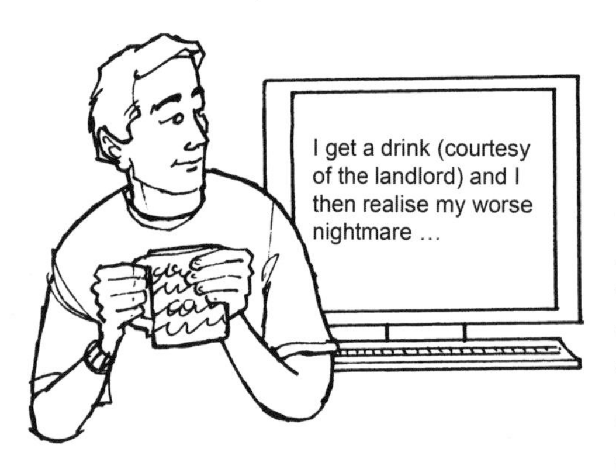

Eventually we decide to go. We arrive at the venue on the dot. I get a big cheer from the rest of the band and the audience. Wow – that feels good. I'm due to join them on stage at 10.15. Annie and I get a drink (courtesy of the landlord) and I then realise my worse nightmare (well second worst). The bag needs emptying. I have to empty the bag in a pub loo (not always in the top rank – except on smell perhaps), five minutes before I'm due on stage. I'm nervous – for the first time in ages. Not just because of the bag, but also because the band has played for the last three months or so without me. Will I fit back in?

The loo is usable and I empty the bag. I get back just as they're calling for me to go on. The audience cheer and clap. This is the best medicine – and it's free. Many friends and acquaintances have made the journey to come and see us. I have to start the first song with a vocal – no instrumental introduction. I get a note for reference and jump straight in. The foldback is great – I can hear myself and it all sounds so good.

I've decided that I'll have to sit down when I play the guitar – it hits the bag when I stand. The last song is up-tempo and I just can't sit down to do it. So I grab the mike and it feels like I've never been away. We do an encore and someone says afterwards *'the jigsaw is complete'.*

I have been looking forward to this moment for so long. In my darkest days in critical care I thought about the things that sustain me – that I can hold on to. And making music with others is one of them. I just love singing. So Good Friday, which turned bad for a while, came good in the end.

Good news? – You tell me

April 22nd 2006

'We looked at your scans this morning; we can confirm that there is only one tumour on your liver. However, we were surprised to find that it is growing much faster than we expected.'

It's only really now that I realise I have Cancer. I've even given it a capital letter to signify that it's a big deal. Although I'm heartened by the news that there is only one tumour, I'm alarmed by the fact that, not only is it growing, but it's doing so at a rate which concerns my doctors. There is more news to come; there may be other malevolent cells around – in fact it's highly likely that cancer cells beyond the resolving power of the scanners are on an insidious journey around my body. The doctor explained the progress of the disease in exponential terms. I have a science degree; I understand exponential growth. This is scary stuff.

Up to this point I've really only thought about the bag and getting over surgery. Although I went through a bad time at Christmas, I got over it fairly quickly and the drama of the operation and life with an ileostomy have consumed all my energy. Now, as I get on with my life – as I write this, even – this thing is growing.

For the first time I'm angry. I've lost two months. The first is due to the bowel join breaking down and is no one's fault. The second month could have been avoided. The request for scans was 'mislaid' and I could have been having this discussion at the end of March instead of the end of April.

Plans have now changed. Surgery is considered inappropriate – too risky. It has a success rate of 35%. I will have a course of chemotherapy as soon as possible, with liver surgery in the autumn. On the positive side this buys me some time – I can try and have a good summer, chemo not withstanding – but a reverse ileostomy is also a major operation and so it'll be 2007 before the bag comes off and I can come off the Homer Simpson diet.

I don't know if it's reasonable to be angry – I know people are doing their best. Would starting chemo a month earlier make any difference? I really don't know. It's partly the way the information is explained that causes anxiety and concern. If I hadn't kept telephoning to get a date for the scans, how much more of a delay would there have been and how much further would the disease have progressed?

Annie and I are both scared; although we are determined to put a positive spin on this, it casts a shadow.

We got home from Oxford about 5pm and the telephone rang. It was Vanessa (one of the specialist nurses in the colorectal unit at Milton Keynes). She has lots of patients to look after and I hadn't seen her for a few weeks, but she remembered I was going to Oxford today and had taken the trouble to ring for news. If you're going to get bowel cancer, MK is the place to get it. As ever, she was brilliant – understood our fears – but optimistic that one tumour is good news. She's offered to chase the oncologist responsible for the chemo regime for me.

So – is it funny hat time? Will I lose my hair and not my beard? If so, will I end up looking like a real-ale drinker or a Morris Dancer? You tell me.

Thar she blows

April 24th 2006

At the beginning of our relationship I was a bit wary, a bit cautious – you know how it is – you want to show interest but you don't want to get let down. I tried to play it cool, but in the end decided to make the effort and in spite of numerous ups and downs we're learning to get along.

There was a big letdown this morning, which just testifies to the strength of the relationship. In the past if this had happened, I'd have shouted and cursed and had a right old sulk. Now I just ride the punches and laugh. Perhaps some of it is my fault anyway because I do take risks with this relationship. Like eating blueberries for breakfast.

It was mid-morning and I was coming downstairs. I felt that old familiar feeling – I raced back up to the bathroom just in time. It was leaking on two sides and going everywhere, down my legs, on my undercarriage and on the loo seat. I used up a whole pack of wipes (which usually lasts me a week) and had to resort to loo paper. Now those who know me well will testify that I can be a bit clumsy. I've thought of making a stage act out of the number of times I've hit my head on a mike when bending down to pick up my guitar.

I had the basin full of water to wipe up the mess. And bear in mind that everything I have to do has to be done one-handed, because I'm trying to stem the flow with the other. I have the loo paper balanced on the basin so that it's within easy reach. In my haste I knock it into the basin and it ends up a sodden, useless mess. I laugh, which is not easy, because at the same time, I have the bottom of my tee shirt and sweatshirt clamped firmly in my teeth to keep them up out of the way. And then it happens – an almighty eruption. An inky black stream of blueberries shoots out of my belly. And goes on and on and on. Where does it all come from? It is bordering on the farcical – I just have to laugh.

All the pictures in the *'you and your stoma'* leaflets show a man naked while changing his bag. Well you wouldn't really take it seriously if he appeared with his pants round his ankles and his top in his teeth. It would distract a bit from the message.

After what seems like minutes there is a break in the flow. I relax — no — thar she blows again. I imagine the blueberries queuing up like paratroopers waiting to jump:

'Wait till he's not looking. He's turning away – no – he's looking back. Wait, wait, wait. Now. Go, Go, Go.'

I don't remember eating that many blueberries. Or is it revenge, stored up anger for all the forbidden fruit I've eaten which has passed quietly and without fuss into the bag? Now I think of it, I took a real risk with a real forbidden fruit last night — blackberry and apple crumble. Well — life's too short.

Eventually there is a lull. I manage to hold a bit of wet loo paper over the spot and get my shoes and pants off with my free hand. I'm out of loo roll now. Don't you just hate it when that happens? I have to find an alternative. It means going downstairs though. So, with my top still clamped in my teeth, the wet loo paper in place — and naked from the waist down — I make my way down stairs. Please, please don't let anyone come to the front door or look through the front window.

The only alternative is kitchen roll. Have you ever tried to tear off a bit of kitchen roll one-handed? I lay the roll down on the kitchen worktop and hold it still with my forehead, while I tear off a couple of sheets with my free hand. I'd pay good money to see this. Let me know if you want tickets.

This sort of thing doesn't really throw me anymore — well not at home. I've learnt to deal with it. I'm still anxious when I go out though. And that's one of the hard things about having a bag — living in an almost permanent state of anxiety. I could play safe and just eat rubbish. But where's the fun in that? Like with all relationships I've had to learn to compromise and so now I don't eat fruit for breakfast if I'm going out for the day. Let that be a lesson to you all.

(un)Easy rider

April 29th 2006

I'm flying down hill, the wind is in my face, the sun is burning into my back – and I'm laughing because I'm riding 'no hands'. Of course it's a fantasy – this is how I imagine it will be. The reality is different in two important respects. The parts about flying down hill, the wind and the sun are all correct. But I'm not laughing and I'm not riding 'no hands' – I'm gritting my teeth and hanging on for grim death.

For the first time since the beginning of January I'm riding my new bike. I've dreamt of doing this for months, but it's not as much fun as I thought – at least not at first. Do I have the energy to do this? Will the bag leak? I'm going to get funny looks (probably worse) if I have to empty it at the side of the road.

My neck and wrists ache. I still need to fiddle around with the position of the bars and stem to make the bike more comfortable (which is not uncommon with a new bike). Annie keeps pulling ahead, but generously waits for me. We're riding round the Redway cycle paths in Milton Keynes. The surface is smooth which keeps the bag relatively quiet. There are over 150 miles of cycle paths in MK but we won't see anything like that distance.

It's warm and I feel the promise of summer in the air. This is one of the joys of riding a bike. Our route includes four hills – or inclines to be more accurate. I manage to ride up each one without having to get off and push (24 gears helps of course). And what goes up must come down – and eventually I do get to the part where I can ride 'no hands'. Yes. I even manage a smile.

Riding a bike always takes me back to my youth when I belonged to a cycling club. I had three bikes then; a racing bike (I managed the odd race or two) a touring bike and a 'going to work on' bike. I thought nothing of riding a 30 mile training circuit with my mates after work – even in the winter – three times a week. I don't think much of it now.

I have two bikes at present – three if I count my old mountain bike which I've converted to a static exercise bike. The new bike is a *Specialized Crossroads Elite* – it's what is called a 'hybrid' – it looks like a mountain bike but has thinner wheels and tyres for riding on the road (as opposed to off-road). Like most bikes these days, it has an aluminium frame and 24 gears and is just the thing for a lazy ride, taking in the sights and smells and sounds.

When I want to go fast, I have a sports bike – drop handlebars, thin wheels and no mudguards. It's a *Kaffenback* – so named because the makers thought it was the ideal bike for riding to the Kaff (café) and back. I'm not making this up. The steel frame is finished in a beautiful blue colour. There's a retro 'steel is real' thing going on in UK bikes circles at the moment. But just to show I'm no Luddite it does have some carbon components. I bought the frame last summer and put the bike together myself as a project. It's my equivalent of a classic sports car – I only take it out when the sun is shining and the roads are dry. There is something about riding a bike with drop handlebars that you don't get from other bikes (apart from a sore neck that is) – the sheer joy and fun of going fast. Each time I take it out I feel a connection with all my heroes of the *Tour de France* – the ones from the 1960s as well as the present. I'm determined to ride it this summer.

We managed 5.5 miles in 47 minutes – an average speed of 7mph. My chest and lungs hurt more than my legs. This was harder than I thought. But I'm encouraged enough to have a go at a cancer charity bike ride in July. It's a 12 mile circuit of MK and is 11 weeks away, so plenty of time to build up for it. I'll be well into chemo by then but hope that doesn't stop me (I wouldn't want to disappoint all my sponsors).

Twelve miles is not far; there was a time when I could ride ten times that distance in a day. At 16 I rode from Guildford to Southampton, a distance of 60 miles, in three hours and ten minutes. It took me a bit longer to ride back. Crossing America is a bit far though. I've just been reading about Jane Tomlinson, a woman with advanced breast cancer, who will shortly cycle across America for charity. She was given six months to live six years ago and is undergoing chemo to keep it at bay. Puts my 12 miles in the shade.

Chemo-savvy

May 5th 2006

And so it begins. A second front in the battle for my body is about to open up. The first salvo of Operation *'Body Storm'* will be fired at 12.00 hours on Tuesday 16th May. Collateral damage is inevitable – innocent bystanders (the good cells) will be destroyed along with the enemy. Just how much collateral damage will occur is unknown. Those cells which divide rapidly – skin, hair, lining of the mouth and digestive system – as well as the cancer cells – are in the front line. At present we cannot simply target the enemy and avoid the civilians – the drugs do not discriminate. Seems to me we need smart weapons instead of weapons of mass destruction.

The day before, at 09.30 hours, a line will be inserted – hopefully into a vein in my arm. If the veins are reluctant to get involved (and who can blame them) then it's to the operating theatre for a line into the chest. Then home to relax until the kick-off.

The current plan is for six cycles of treatment once a fortnight. A cocktail of drugs will be injected and then the big one will drip into my body over a 48-hour period. Fortunately the drug can be administered by a pump, which I will wear (somehow) – this means I don't have to stay in hospital, but can come home while the battle rages. So, another dinky medical accessory to add to my collection.

Meet the troops at the Oncology Centre at Northampton this morning. A staff nurse shows me around the battlefield – a group of a dozen or so reclining chairs arranged in a sort of horse-shoe shape. Could be mistaken for a furniture showroom – except the white pillow on the right arm of each chair says that this is no ordinary gathering of furniture. This is where I'll spend the first two hours of each 48 having cocktails. The staff seem very nice and there are other patients getting dosed up. Everyone looks so normal – you wouldn't pick them out in the street as needing chemo.

I leave with a little green book which details my treatment, lists side-effects, and emergency numbers to contact. There's a lot to take in.

I need a blood test the day before each cycle. The pump has to be disconnected (in hospital) at the end of each 48-hour cycle and the line flushed out once a week. I'm provided with a supply of anti-nausea drugs but I'll need to get a thermometer to monitor my temperature (over 38°C means an infection). The blood tests are essential for gauging the effect on my bone marrow. If the blood count falls between cycles, the next may be delayed to give them time to recover. I'm going to have to start eating red meat – particularly liver (the irony of eating liver to save my own is not lost on me) or start drinking stout instead of cider.

It's a full-time job having cancer – there's a lot to learn and a lot to do. You have to become sensitive to minute changes in your body, without becoming a hypochondriac. You have to know your enemy if you want to defeat it. So there's a lot of research to do – on the progress of the disease and the treatments available. I could really do with a PA.

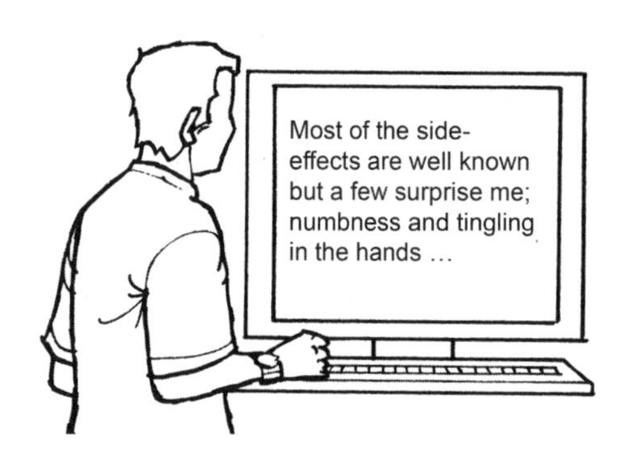

Most of the side-effects are well known but a few surprise me; numbness and tingling in the hands – not a big deal you might think, but could make playing the guitar difficult – and it's not unknown to drop a cold drink taken from the fridge. Another is more scary – laryngeal spasm – affecting the voice box. Again it's related to low temperatures; so even if I manage to hang on to a cold drink from the fridge, I shouldn't drink it – especially not before a gig. And then there's depression; in fact depression is now seen as a side-effect of cancer itself, not just chemo. So it's perfectly normal to feel low with this disease. Which is a relief.

Having said that, many of the side-effects are rare. And that's the odd thing – some people will experience a number of side-effects, some people will get a few and some may get none at all.

The next 12 weeks or so are going to be eventful, one way or another. I want to fit in a couple of gigs and a charity bike ride. It looks as if the chemo cycles will be on Tuesdays, which means my weekends should be fine. I'll report back in my next dispatches from the front.

So far so good

May 15th 2006

There's one thing I now know that I cannot do one-handed – empty my bag. This realisation dawns as I sit waiting for an X-ray at Northampton Hospital. The bag is dangerously full and my left arm is bandaged from the wrist to above the elbow. It is also straight as a die – no chance of bending it. It's a substantial bandage – my arm looks like the sort a mummy would have in one of those mummy horror films. In fact, if ever there is an opening for a stand-in left arm in any such film, I'll audition.

I'm getting anxious – both about the perilous state of the bag and the results of the X-ray. I should have paid more attention when I came for a blood test at the Oncology Centre at Northampton last week. X-ray was vaguely mentioned – or rather it was mentioned, but I vaguely heard it. The reason I'm waiting for an X-ray is that I've had a line inserted in my arm but the end of it could be in one of two places. It should have reached my chest, but it could have taken a wrong turn – perhaps gone the pretty way – and ended up in my neck. I collect the X-ray film and make my way back to the oncology unit to find out the results.

The insertion of the line – a PICC line (Peripherally Inserted Central Catheter) – is a remarkable thing. Again, I'm glad I didn't pay too much attention last week when the process was explained. Sometimes ignorance is bliss. I do remember the nurse saying that the needle was bigger than the sort they use for IV drips and blood tests, but I would be given anaesthetic gel to rub on my arm to numb the pain.

Now when she said 'bigger' I assumed she was referring to the diameter – ie., it would be fatter than normal. What she meant was longer – about 50cm longer as it turns out. I finally realised that this was quite a big deal when I was taken over to a bed to lie on and the nurse who would perform the procedure started to put on her scrubs.

As the line went in the nurse delivered a running commentary to her audience; me, a trainee nurse in attendance and a senior nurse holding my arm and muttering words of comfort. It appeared to be going in just fine – she squealed with delight as it progressed up my arm, round my shoulder and ... where next however, was anyone's guess. She was doing this blind – the line is calibrated so she can see how far it has gone in – but she cannot tell where it has ended up. Hence the X-ray.

Thankfully the line had arrived at my chest (*'I'm so pleased'* she said – over and over – so much so that I asked her if this was the first one she'd done. She reassured me that she'd done this procedure over 200 times, but simply wanted me to have some luck for a change). As it turned out, it had not gone in far enough. A doctor confirmed that it needed to go in another 4cm – so that it would come to rest beside the 4th rib. So, she gently pushed the line in again and total distance travelled finished up at 52cm. A completely painless procedure.

I was warned that my body might try and reject the line and to watch for swelling and pain overnight. By the time I got back to Milton Keynes, it had started to bleed through the dressing. A quick visit to the Macmillan Unit at MK hospital reassured me that this was normal – and could be left until tomorrow when I start the chemo. And to complete the story, once all the bandages had come off – they were there simply to protect my arm while I went for an X-ray – I was able to bend my arm a little and so empty my bag. A happy ending then.

How are you? Well actually ...

May 16th 2006

I knew this would happen. I'd been thinking about what I'd say when the situation eventually arose. But I couldn't settle on the most appropriate response. And sure enough, four times in the past two weeks I've met people I'd not seen for years. I'd rehearsed three responses to the inevitable greeting '*How are you*?'

1. *'Well actually I have advanced bowel cancer.'*
2. *'How do I look?'*
3. *'Just fine – how are you?'*

Annie was with me when I had the opportunity to try out the first. We met someone in a supermarket checkout that I used to work with. He was visibly shocked by my response, so much so that Annie was concerned for *'that poor man'* as we made our way home.

I've always assumed honesty was the best policy. I want to let people know so that they have a chance to work out a response that does not cause embarrassment or awkwardness. Very easy to do by email. Much more difficult face-to-face.

I find it difficult to deliver the second response without sounding confrontational — which is not my intention at all. It's merely a device to open the conversation. This one went down reasonably well, but that may have had as much to do with the other person as me.

I briefly considered a variation on the second: *'Do you really want to know?'* There is no way of saying that without sounding aggressive. I quickly abandoned the idea.

The third response is the classic British understatement and should not be taken at face value. It is simply a form of greeting — a variation on *'good morning'* and has nothing to do with an interest in the other person's health.

There is one thing though that face-to-face can do rather well; the way the line is delivered can let the other person know immediately whether I have a positive or a negative attitude to the disease. I have to sprinkle a few jokes or asides in an email (which the recipient may or may not get) in order to convey the fact that I see cancer as an inconvenience rather than anything else. And those who have read all my blogs will know that my biggest battle is with the *****!!!!! ***** bag.

When I had the line put in, the nurse asked if I wanted a gauze sleeve to put over my arm in case I was worried about people seeing it. I declined the offer – I'm not at all embarrassed about it. It was only driving home that I realised that this was as much about other people as it was about me. The line exits from the crook of my elbow and with the various attachments reaches down to my wrist. We're fast approaching tee-shirt weather and soon it will be very visible. Maybe people going to one of our gigs, out for a good time, don't want their evening spoiled by a reminder of the darker side of life. On the other hand, I want to show people that cancer need not stop you getting on with your life. It's a tricky one.

One down – five to go

May 16th – 18th 2006

Tuesday May 16th

I decided about 15 years or so ago that I would not offer unsolicited advice. This resolution came after listening to an American management guru (can't recall his name – but he used to be a big cheese in the Xerox Corp) – tell a group of UK managers *'whoever said it is better to give than to receive, was not talking about advice'.* That pearl of wisdom has stayed with me ever since and I've tried hard not to go back on it. Until today. As the chemo regime gets underway I feel bound to pass one nugget on – asked for or not.

I could, of course, say that someone had asked for advice – it's an old trick that musicians use when they run out of songs at a gig. They just start from the beginning again, saying that some members of the audience arrived late and have requested these songs. It usually works. I should add that *Fat Freddy's Cat* never resorts to this sort of deception.

As I sit in the comfy chair at the Oncology Centre in Northampton, a nurse struggles to remove a dressing that encases my left forearm. It's quite a tricky job because the hairs on my arm are pulling and distending the skin around where the line goes in. There's been a small amount of bleeding overnight around the entry point that needs cleaning away to prevent infection. Having removed the dressing the nurse then tries to shave my arm without disturbing the line: *'We really should have done this before we started'.*

If I had a pound coin for every time I've heard this, I'd be able to afford the hospital car park fees.

So this is it; if you're contemplating any surgical procedure, no matter how minor (or major) have a good shave first. In fact go the whole hog and have a full body wax. We all know that pulling plasters off hairy bodies hurts – and we also know that women do this on a regular basis and that they're much braver than men. But that's beside the point. It's not just about the fact that it hurts. Hairs also prevent things sticking properly to the skin. When I had the 'abnormal heart arrhythmia' episode, I needed an ECG. This had to be done twice – the sensors wouldn't stick to my chest until after it had been shaved. And changing the dressings (daily) on my stomach wound was particularly painful as it had not healed and all the tugging and pulling only seemed to make it worse. In each case the nurse involved would stop and go off and look for a razor before continuing. Even the bag sometimes leaks because the hairs around the stoma prevent it sticking properly and on my routine visits to the Bag Lady she ends up playing the role of barber. So there you have it. It's better done before, than during. Of course, if you're challenged in the body hair department then I guess it's less of a problem. But I digress.

Getting to Northampton was quite a challenge in itself. The Centre advised against me driving myself for the first session as my reaction to the drugs would be unknown. The whole procedure takes about three hours or so and I didn't want Annie sitting there twiddling her thumbs when she could be attempting to lever quadratic equations into young minds intent on resisting such overtures. I'll be finished by the time school ends and she'll be able to collect me. So her eldest, Chris, takes me in his brand new Audi A4 (*Good grief are we there already?*) Quattro. It's a nice car finished in a sinister shade of black, but as the fields and villages of Northamptonshire fly by, I begin to wonder what effect the G-forces might have on the stoma bag – and in particular what the bag might do to the new leather upholstery. In the event, nothing – we arrive 20 minutes early – bag intact.

I while away the time in the waiting room playing 'spot the patient'. Most of the others are in couples and they're all older than me. It's hard to tell who is getting the chemo and who is the supporter. A lonely headscarf provides a possible clue. A gentleman sitting near me gets up and goes to the loo and his wife leans across and asks if I'm here for the chemo. I nod and she volunteers that her husband has completed his treatment and is waiting to find out the next stage (so an easy one to spot there – no points awarded). When he returns I find out he also has bowel cancer with four tumours on his liver and will need around three quarters of the liver removed. I am still amazed when I hear these stories. The liver is clearly a remarkable organ, to grow back after such an assault. I resolve to treat mine with much more respect in future and drink only at weekends. Apart from my medicinal Guinness that is.

There are three other patients in the chemotherapy treatment room by the time I'm called in. One is asleep but the other two start chatting. I'm told that the side effects really kick in around session four. They mean well but as I listen I discover we all have different cancers and hence are on different drugs, so the effects may not be universal. I hope not as I have a charity bike planned just after session five.

The first drug takes two hours to administer and I tuck in to my lunch. I was advised to bring food and drink – this has much the same effect as eating on a long haul flight, but also militates against any side effects, particularly nausea. My mind begins to wander and I try to think of a collective noun for chemo patients. I give up at my first attempt – chemo-holics and doze off.

I ate very little before I set off for Northampton, which given I was to be there for three hours, turned out to be a good move as it meant the bag would not require emptying while I was there. Although it is possible to go to the loo while connected up to the drip (it's on wheels) the lead is not long enough to allow for the full dexterity needed for bag-work.

The second drug takes just 15 minutes and then the line is flushed with a saline solution. I feel OK so far apart from a general tiredness. Annie arrives as I'm being connected up to my pump. It's battery operated, and about the size of a baby's feeding bottle. I'm given a pouch to hang round my neck and a supply of drugs to take home to combat the effects of chemo: steroids, a strong anti-nausea drug, some mild anti-nausea drugs and boxes of Imodium. It seems that the chemo and the steroids loosen everything up and the anti-nausea and Imodium slow everything down. It all seems a bit excessive – a 'belt and braces' approach. But I may yet have cause to be grateful.

By the time we get home the bag needs emptying and the short-comings of the pouch become apparent. Without going into too much detail, it simply gets in the way. I find an old bum-bag (fanny-pack to my American friends) and this provides a better solution. A shoulder holster of the type beloved by American cops would be ideal – and look rather cool.

As evening comes I start to feel extremely tired. Wearing the pump in bed proves awkward, the line is too short (or I'm too tall), to fit under the pillow as suggested and I end up sleeping on my back with it next to me. I drop off to my usual night-time incantation *'Please don't let the bag leak, please don't let the bag leak'.* I say it with more feeling this time – if it does leak I'll need at least four hands this time instead of the three ideally required to change the bag.

Wednesday May 17th

I wake early feeling a little nauseous. A slice of toast and a pill should do the trick. I get some bread from the freezer to make toast and experience the tingling fingers from the cold bread. This is weird. Could have been scary had I not known to expect it.

Later on I decide to conduct a scientific experiment – to see if eating ice cream brings on laryngeal spasm (you can tell I'm bored). I wear gloves this time as I get a tub of *Ben & Jerry's* Fish Food from the freezer. Interestingly (and thankfully) no ill effects – but the taste is completely different – bitter and unpleasant in fact. In the interests of medical research I decide to make a comparison with vanilla ice cream. This tastes normal. So it's chocolate flavoured ice cream that's affected by the chemo drugs. Hmm.

Thursday May 18th

No obvious feeling of nausea on waking this morning. Decide to change bag first thing. Lucky I did so as it was close to leaking. This happened yesterday at about the same time.

As I type this mid-morning I get a major leak. I'm just sitting here at the computer – no undue movement to disturb the bag. It's bad enough to require a dip in the bath afterwards to clean myself up. This is really hard – I have to sling the pump round my neck, while keeping a bit of kitchen roll over the stoma to contain it, as I ferret around in my bag looking for wipes, new stoma bag and so on. I hate to think how someone less agile than me would cope with all this. Still, it keeps my mind off cancer.

Lunchtime – and it goes again – this is a record. It's really getting me down now. It's not just the mess; it's all the fiddling around trying to cope one-handed. I call the Bag Lady for advice. She asks me to come in to MK hospital straightaway. (How's that for service?) I'm her only patient with this problem at present – which should be a comfort to others with an ileostomy. She's concerned that I'm not going to get through chemo at this rate. She brings out the heavy guns – a super-bag held in place by both adhesive and a belt. The belt is uncomfortable but I agree to give it a go – at least while I'm on chemo. Leaks are far, far worse. I guess I'll have to try Imodium as well or give up coffee and fruit for the duration.

The pump comes off late afternoon. I feel an immense sense of relief and freedom.

By late evening I have a chance to reflect on the past two days. Overall

I feel OK. I have to get the bag sorted out though – the drugs are clearly messing with the digestive system. The pump is a nuisance – I can't shower with it attached – and sleeping, and dealing with the bag, is awkward. But it does mean I don't have to spend two nights in hospital, which is a fair trade. I guess I'll get used to it. That's the first session over – only five more to go.

Three steps forwards – two steps back

May 26th 2006

It's been a long week. I've had plenty of time on my hands. Annie's been decorating and I've not, I've just been too tired. My left arm, where the line has gone in, has been sore and swollen and I've needed analgesics for pain relief. I haven't been able to lift the arm above my shoulder. This was all to be expected and shouldn't last more than 'a few days'.

The effects of the first chemo session have also made themselves felt. It starts in the mouth. Nothing tastes as it should – food, drink – it's all just, well ... bleugh. Even my brain is affected as I run out of appropriate adjectives. My digestive system has been more 'stop-go' than the British Economy of the 70s. I have not experienced nausea as such – just an indefinable sense that something is 'not quite right'.

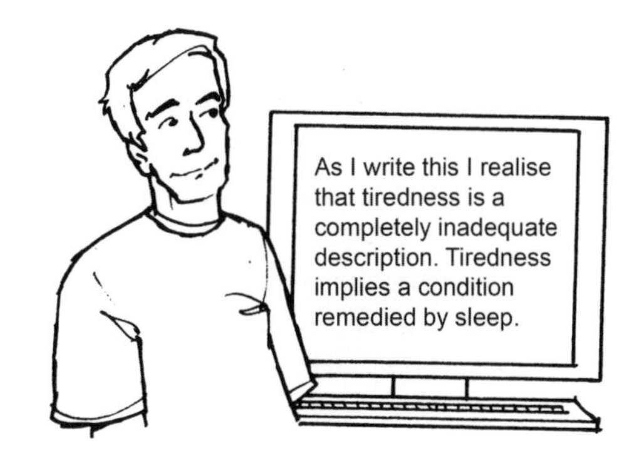

Above all, it's the tiredness. As I write this I realise that tiredness is a completely inadequate description. Tiredness implies a condition remedied by sleep. This is not the case – sleep does not help. Perhaps it's more a weariness, because it affects me mentally as well as physically. I just can't concentrate for very long; reading or playing the guitar takes a lot of effort. And as for watching television ...

I've heard from a number of people who've been through chemotherapy and it seems to affect people in different ways. But what is common is this feeling of tiredness/weariness/exhaustion. I am humbled by chemo – in particular by the fact that describing it accurately has defeated me.

It's reminiscent of the period when I first returned home from hospital. It's not as bad as that – I can do far more now than I could then. But I feel I've taken a retrograde step. I've had to cancel two gigs this coming weekend and I missed an old friend's wedding last Saturday. This was particularly galling as Annie had bought a new outfit and I was looking forward to trying out the new bag under my faithful, expandable Rohans. On the positive side though, the new super bag seems to be doing the trick and I've finished the first course of steroids. So no more Mr Grumpy.

The district nurse has just been to flush out the line with a saline solution and to change the dressing. This is something that needs to be done once a week. It turned out to be my original nurse and I was really pleased to see him again. The line is not stitched in, thank goodness, but held in place by four very small tape dressings. He carefully and gently lifted each of these and cleaned away the dried blood that had seeped from the line entry. He did this without causing me any pain or discomfort. This has made a difference to how I feel and today, for the first time since starting chemo, it seems as if I'm moving forwards again, albeit slowly.

It's not really productive time that I have available. I keep thinking I should do something useful like fill in my tax return. But that's now been simplified and isn't going to keep me occupied for long.

One thing I can do is to prepare the stoma bags for when they need changing – (it's not all fun and games with a stoma – there is work to do as well). This means cutting a hole in the back to match the shape of my stoma. I try to do a week's supply in one go. I learnt the hard way that you cannot take the old one off and then try and cut a hole in a new one. The stoma changes in shape and diameter over time and the correct size of hole is based on a template measured by the Bag Lady. I have not yet got to the stage where I can manage this for myself.

As I cut out a hole I take a long hard look at the new stoma bag. With its mouth open it looks a bit like a lamprey – it wouldn't look out of place in the ocean stuck to the side of some poor unsuspecting sea creature. Well it would for obvious reasons, but life's too short to worry about the suitability of a metaphor.

There is a lot to this bag. The adhesive pad is thicker and much harder to get off than the old one – I imagine eight pints and a Vindaloo would not shift it. The Bag Lady has given me a few to try out and as it seemed to be so successful – one week, no leak – I log on to the Internet to order more. And this is a revelation. There's a whole world of surgical appliances out there that seems to have passed me by. I had no idea there were so many bag designs. I can see stoma care taking over from computers, football and DIY as the natural subject for male discourse:

bloke 1: *'I see you've got the new Pelico Super-Convex, Velcro Twin with triple-fold exhaust.'*

bloke 2: *'Well it's the natural upgrade over the Dansak Velcro Single. And the belt, as well as being functional, has a real retro look to it.'*

bloke 1: *'Oh yeah – I like 1950s NHS spectacle pink. That bit of sticky tape is a nice touch.'*

bloke 2: *'I just got to the stage where I started to wonder – what am I doing with my life? The kids have left home, it's just me and the old bag now, so I thought – what the heck – I've always wanted to try a Velcro Twin ...'*

I sometimes wonder (another consequence of too much time on my hands) why I got cancer. The conclusion I'm forced to is that it's just bad luck. Neither of my parents had bowel cancer and, although two daughters of a cousin succumbed to the disease in their early 30s (tragically both leaving behind young families) I think these instances too remote to suggest any genetic predisposition.

I've always tried to eat a healthy diet. I mentioned to the Bag Lady one day that perhaps I should stop eating red meat, given that some researchers suggest a link between red meat and bowel cancer. She said that over 25% of her patients are vegetarians and that I should not worry and eat what I enjoy. This started me thinking about junk food. I've come to the conclusion that there is no such thing as junk food – only a junk diet. I lose a lot of salt from my system as a consequence of the ileostomy and so crisps, and other various salty snacks, have become, for the time being, an essential part of my diet.

For the past ten years I have taken my dog out for a walk twice a day in all weathers, walked to work when I could and ridden my bike for fun and exercise. Playing in a band is better than a gym – a two-hour gig gives a full bodywork out; lifting gear and singing exercises both lungs and muscles. So I consider myself to be reasonably fit. And apart from a couple of minor hiccups like divorce and redundancy, I've had a charmed life stress-wise. Not really a strong case for environmental or lifestyle causes. So I'm left with *happenstance* (love that word) or *kismet* (that too) or any other variation on the basic idea that *'stuff happens'*.

I rather like the idea that my cancer is simply bad luck. It means there is no person or circumstance to blame. Which means I have no regrets about the life I lead. Which, in turn, makes me happy. Not smug mind you, just happy with my lot.

An unwelcome visitor

June 11th 2006

Chemo is getting me down and I'm having to work hard to remain positive. The second cycle started on May 31st. I won't go on about how tired it makes me feel – that's a given. A few bizarre things have happened though. On day two I had a spasm in my throat when I got a cold drink from the fridge. It feels like my throat is swelling up with shards of ice and I'm not going to be able to breathe – and then it goes as quickly as it came. The really weird thing is that the throat doesn't actually swell up – it just feels as if it is. The same day my right thumb locked itself to the palm of my right hand. I couldn't move it for about five minutes.

The nausea is worse this time. It arrives unannounced each day like an unwelcome visitor. I can be just sitting around minding my own business and suddenly there it is – invading my space. There's nothing much I can do except take the pills and wait for it to go. It only lasted about five days or so after the first cycle. This time it's been twelve days – the next one starts in two days time and I've had virtually no respite in between.

If it carries on like this – and the side-effects are expected to be cumulative – then I'm not going to be able to do some of the things I planned to do in between. One thing I have pencilled in is a Cancer Research bike ride in July. I considered buying some new carbon forks for my racing bike – and then thought *'Why bother – I may not get to ride it again'*. I have to put this remark in context: I've just been reading about someone with bowel cancer who went through chemo to shrink the tumours on his liver – the tumours did indeed shrink – but then grew back and he died. He was only a couple of years older than me. I'm not simply feeling sorry for myself – this is the new reality. I may go through all this for nothing. Having said all that, boredom, the Internet and my credit card eventually came to the rescue and the carbon forks are on their way as I write this (phew – close call).

I had a card from my ex-sister-in-law[2] saying that she wept with laughter at my last blog – and then felt guilty for laughing at my misfortune. My view is *'If in doubt – laugh'*. From the moment I first went into hospital I could see a funny side to all this. I guess if it didn't make me laugh, it would probably make me cry. The problem right now is that I cannot find a funny side to chemo. I've looked really hard, but it's just nowhere to be found. Perhaps it got zapped along with my cells.

Annie has not lost her sense of humour, fortunately. She suggests I apply to go on *Big Brother* – she thinks *'I'm just off to empty my bag'* would keep the nation glued to their TV sets. The district nurse has not lost his sense of humour either. He took off all the old dressings, cleaned up the area around the line in my arm and then, as he prepared to put on the new dressings, said, *'If you want to scratch, now would be a good time'* – well it made me laugh.

A few days ago my watch stopped. As someone who feels undressed without a wristwatch, I find an old one to use in the meantime. It was the first thing I ever bought when I left school and started work 43 years ago. It's clockwork rather than electronic and just needs winding up to go. Although it's a bit grubby, it works and is in marginally better shape than I am after all this time, although – like me – it does keep slowing down.

The new bag is also working like clockwork with no leaks in three weeks. Given the effort that the bag has made to behave itself, I am now prepared to meet it halfway and I feel we're entering a new phase in our relationship. I might even get to like it (only joking).

It was my birthday yesterday and Annie took me out for breakfast. The restaurant was on the first floor and I was out of breath from climbing one flight of stairs. The band had a gig in the evening and I was due to play the second set, but I did begin to wonder if I'd have the energy. I rested in the afternoon – the England-Paraguay match providing the perfect excuse to get some sleep. Around 7.00pm the unwelcome visitor returned. I took a couple of pills and sat it out. I was still feeling low when I arrived at the gig, but I had a great time. Everyone tells me how well I look; someone said that I looked yellow and drawn when I first arrived but was positively glowing by the end.

I'm still on a high when we arrive home – with my optimism duly returned and my credit card still beside my computer, I decide to treat myself to a new watch. Now if this next one were to last 43 years – that really would be something.

[2] I hate that phrase – *ex* has such negative connotations. Marion always has been, and always will be, my sister. It's not her and I that got divorced. As our society changes we're going to have to come up with better words to describe these types of relationships.

Halfway to paradise

June 15th 2006

It's only when I put my foot down on the M1 that my mood begins to lift. I've decided to drive myself to chemo. The effects don't kick in until well after the session is finished so I feel quite safe to drive home again. It's a sense of freedom that I badly need. I feel as if I've been imprisoned for much of the past two weeks with just a couple of days off for good behaviour.

My mood lifts further when I read a newspaper article claiming that cycling is the fastest and easiest way to regain fitness (I'm at the hospital now in case you think I'm reading the newspaper while driving). I'm inspired to do more when I'm finally free of all this. I have visions of an epic ride – Land's End to John O'Groats perhaps or even The Channel to the Mediterranean. Whose knows? I'll be happy enough to ride my 12-mile circuit of MK without needing a week in bed right now.

This is my third chemo cycle and I'm halfway through. I have this vision of a place – in my head more than geographical – where the drugs have finally left my body in peace and I have a couple of months of no discomfort – where I can get back to some sort of normality before the next stage in my treatment. I would never have guessed six months ago that normal could be paradise. Or rather – that paradise could be found in ordinariness.

I take my *iPod* this time and then have a surreal moment. While the drugs make their way round my bloodstream, I listen to *Rubber Soul* – the irony of both the performers and the listener on drugs is not lost. When I hear George Harrison's sitar, I'm taken back to the 'Summer of Love' – except that *Rubber Soul* came out in 1965 and the 'Summer of Love' was 1967.

In 1965 I had just moved from being paid weekly to a monthly salary with its disastrous consequences on my cash flow – not easy for a teenager. I had to go through a couple of weeks of delicious anticipation before I could finally buy the album. I realise, as I listen and think back, that this was probably the first step – unconscious at the time – in a long transition from working class to middle class – deferred gratification. Back then the idea of sacrifice now for future benefit was one of the defining indicators of middle class life. For my parents there was always hire purchase – or live now-pay later. Although this was in the days before plastic money, so I'm not so sure that distinction holds anymore.

To be fair, my parents were always nagging me to save money – this was more because my father was disabled and unable to work through much of my teenage years, and not because they had aspirations to move up the social ladder. When my father was working, Friday night was treat night. He would bring my mother a box of chocolates on the way home from work and then after tea he and I would walk to the off-licence for a bottle of cider and three packets of crisps – the ones with the little blue waxed bag of salt. I would be about ten years old I guess.

Having finally acquired the habit of squirrelling away nuts for the winter, I also realise that I'm about to come full circle, which raises a dilemma. One of the defining indicators of living with cancer is to live for the moment *'Life's too short – you never know what's round the corner'* – much like the live now-pay later philosophy from my childhood. Because for many cancer patients, there will not be a 'later'. But for many there will be. And the dilemma is this; do I spend all my hard-earned cash now having a good time ... just in case? Or do I save it all for later ... just in case?

It's not just about money – it's also the plans Annie and I have for the future. I know we all have to live with a degree of uncertainty in our lives, but it is this perpetual state of uncertainty that I find the hardest aspect of living with cancer. It'll be years before I know if the disease is in remission. Even though I am positive and determined, positive thinking can be exhausting. And, it has to be said, does not always work. I looked at the five-day weather forecast at the weekend. The prediction was for a sunny, hot week. As I was likely to be spending much of this week dozing off the effects of chemo, I bought a sun-lounger on Saturday. It arrived on Tuesday along with the rain.

Rubber Soul finishes and so does my reminiscence. It's amazing where a couple of hours in a comfy chair hooked up to a machine can lead. I switch off the *iPod* – I've had enough time-travel for one day.

At the end of the session the pump is connected and I'm free to go home. For a moment I feel like a re-offender, a recidivist – the ball and chain will ensure I don't go far in the next 48 hours. But as I drive home with Bruce Springsteen's *Waiting On A Sunny Day* at full blast, I realise I'm smiling.

Happy days

June 23rd 2006

A scientist at the University of Cardiff has announced that, after much research, Friday June 23rd is the happiest day of the year. Well – I'm in a good mood so he must be right.

The chemo drugs have declared a sort of unofficial ceasefire. The mornings are fine and I feel able to get out and about and do things. But just to let me know that they've not gone soft on me, they sneak up around late afternoon and resume hostilities. BUT – and it's a big but – it's not every day they do this.

Apart from getting more respite this time, there are other reasons to be cheerful. The sun is shining, the birds are singing and the postman's just been. The carbon forks for my racing bike have arrived along with my new watch. The forks are so cool – I can't decide whether to put them on the bike or hang them on the wall as an artwork. The watch is also pretty cool – it's based on the 'Official Swiss Railways Watch' – a classic minimalist design and not a cuckoo in sight.

Spending money means I'm going to have to go back to work before too long – partly because my sick pay will run out soon and also because I'm losing touch with the world of work. And also because it's too easy, on the days when I can't do much, to shop on the internet. My plan is to go back to work between the chemo finishing and the liver surgery. I've been off for almost six months and I'm not sure how easy it will be to settle back into the routine and the politics of a large organisation. I keep thinking I ought to do something useful – like the tea ladies who volunteer their services at the hospital. Anyone brought up on a diet of post-war British films will understand the significance of a cup of tea in moments of crisis.

Hmm – this talk of work and the sun's just gone behind a big dark cloud. Well Dr Scientist – what do you think of that? Does your hypothesis still hold? In the interests of science I'll go into the garden and perform a sun dance. This is a traditional British custom involving a barbeque, an umbrella (just in case), copious bottles of beer and the ritual cremation of a sausage. There is no bloodletting – the sausage of choice will generally be of the anaemic variety. And it usually does the trick. As the smoke rises and the sausage passes over to the other side, even the grumpiest, unhappiest male (because it usually is a male in charge of this ceremony) is forced to smile at the satisfaction of a job well done. So – a triumph for science over superstition?

The fact of the matter

June 30th 2006

A fact is something that ultimately defies argument – although what actually constitutes a fact is often the cause of many disagreements. The speed of light is a fact. That the internal angles of a triangle add up to 180° is another – but only up to a point. In a Newtonian Universe this is true. But when the triangle becomes large – and I mean really BIG – as in distances between, say, galaxies – the internal angles add up to more that 180°. Or so I was taught at university. And when the triangle becomes really small as in a nano universe (and I'm not talking *iPods* here) the internal angles are less than 180°. I have no idea why this is the case because I started looking out of the window at this point. I remember something about the curvature of space, but I had my mind on other curves at the time.

It's easy to confuse facts with beliefs. They need a context if they're to make any sense. You can argue about facts – and resolve the dispute because they can be proved, eventually, one way or another. But you cannot argue about beliefs – well you can try, but you're flogging a dead horse because it's very difficult to get people to change long held beliefs.

I realise that I know only one fact about cancer – that it's a life changing disease. I find everything else confusing. Some people react badly to chemo, others don't. Some people will survive the disease, others will not. We hear about 90-year-olds who are fit as a fiddle on a diet of 40 fags a day, and 40-year-olds who succumb to lung cancer having never smoked in their lives.

I guess this is why there is so much emphasis on positive thinking. In the absence of facts, it's a belief to hang on to. I don't know if it works – but I'm reading a book[3] in which the author (a cancer surgeon who has 'evolved' into a cancer therapist) states that medical staff are more likely to do more for a patient with a positive outlook than one who is negative – simply because of human nature. I think there's more to it than that. Those working in healthcare are trained to save lives – it's their *raison d'être* – and are not trained (until recently perhaps) to deal with the end of life. Which is why some terminally ill people die in pain and without dignity. Not so with cancer, it appears – a recent survey shows that over 90% of relatives report their loved ones died a 'good death' – i.e. without pain and with dignity intact. This drops to around 50% for those with chronic lung disease or heart disease[4].

There's a major difference in the timelines for these diseases. Cancer patients, with the appropriate treatment, can appear to lead a 'normal life' – a graph of deterioration over time would be horizontal, before dropping down quite quickly. A similar graph for chronic lung disease, for example, would show a steady decline over the entire timescale. So I guess it's a lot easier to appear positive if your life appears 'normal' than if you're fighting for breath every time you speak.

It's not just the patient whose life is changed by cancer – those around find their lives change too. Apart from Annie, perhaps the biggest change was felt by my dog. I miss him a lot, but took the painful decision to re-home him when I became ill. Although he would have helped in my recovery – I used to walk him every day – I could not have coped with looking after him. He would want to sit on my lap the moment I sat down and my lap was not a good place to be – and still isn't all the time I have the bag. I was lucky to find someone who could give him a good home and although I'd really like to see him again, I know that would be unfair as he's happy and settled. Perhaps not everything that changes is for the worse.

One of my blog entries upset Helen (my step-daughter) because I mentioned the 'D' word (her term for it) – and now I've done it again. Do I sanitise what I write and feel for the sake of others, or do I write the truth – albeit a truth while under the influence of medication? I try to write about the dark side of this disease in a straightforward, unsentimental or self-pitying way because that's the only way I can deal with it. Stuff happens – and we have to get on with it.

I've heard cancer described as living under a sentence of death. I think it's more like being on Death Row. Prisoners can spend over 20 years on Death Row – living in hope for the call from the State Governor with the reprieve. Not only that – their time is spent in solitary confinement, which leads to another similarity. The terminally ill can live in solitary confinement – at least in their heads – because there are some things which are taboo and too difficult to discuss, particularly with those who are closest. This was brought home to me by a recent episode of *Without a Trace* (an American drama series about the FBI's missing persons squad). Although harrowing – this particular missing person was a cancer patient whose treatment was not working – it was tackled with great sensitivity. At its heart was the dilemma faced by the patient in not being able to tell her family that she was going to die because she was trying to protect them – it then went on to deal with the conflict between what the patient wanted (to die in peace) and what the family wanted (for her to carry on fighting). At one point she cries out; *'I'm tired. I don't want to be positive any more'*. I bet she's not the only one.

I've just received a copy of a report sent from my consultant to my employer regarding my prospects for returning to work. Although I have a pretty good idea about what is happening to me it's still a shock to see it written down. My cancer is classed as *Dukes (D)* – a scale running from A-D, which indicates the spread of the disease from its original site. I didn't know it was a D. The report contains the following:

'The long-term prognosis is guarded, but I hope with surgical clearance and vigorous follow up the prospect of a long term cure is possible.'

So 'possible' rather than 'probable'. Perhaps that's the best any of us can hope for. I remain positive – most of the time. And when I'm not, I realise it's just the chemo drugs messing with my mind – and that's a fact.

[3] *Love, Medicine and Miracles*; Bernie S. Seigel, 1986.
[4] *How to have a Good Death*; BBC2 March 31st 2006.

Oh what a beautiful morning

July 7th 2006

Sometimes when I wake up I just want to sing.

There's a bright golden lump on my liver
There's a bright golden lump on my liver
My blood count is high
I'm not gonna die
'Cos the one on my colon is waving goodbye

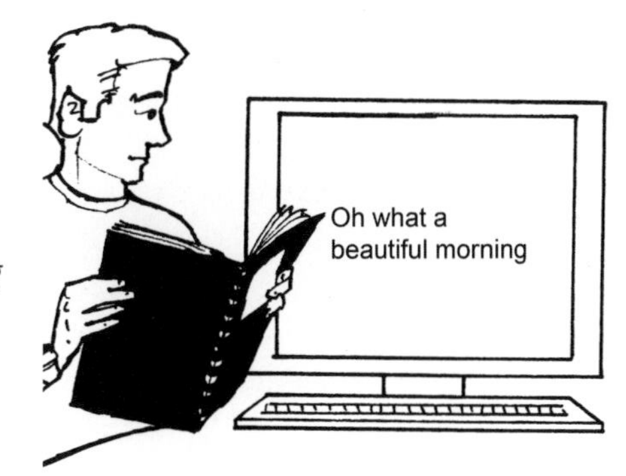

(altogether now..)
Oh what a beautiful morning
Oh what a beautiful day
I've got a beautiful feeling
My cancer is going away

Oh the nurses all smile when they greet me
Oh the nurses all smile when they greet me
I smile but can't speak
'Cos I still feel a freak
With this thing on my stomach that's threatening to leak

Oh what a beautiful morning
Oh what a beautiful day
I've got a beautiful feeling
My cancer is going away

Oh the chemo it does do my head in
Oh the chemo it does do my head in
My tongue is the pits
And I'm covered in zits
But I'm high 'cos my blog has had 22,728[5] *hits*

Oh what a beautiful morning
Oh what a beautiful day
I've got a beautiful feeling
My cancer is going away
Oh what a beautiful day

(Apologies to Rogers and Hammerstein)

I love the song – I don't know whether it will catch on though. That's great news, well done with the blog we've been with you all the way, and today really is a beautiful day. Good on ya mate.

GandM
8th July 2006

[5] And rising…

Chemo 5 – NHS 0

July 11th 2006

I try hard not to complain. I know people are doing their best. But as the great American management guru W. Edwards Deming once said (to me, as it happens, but that's another story) *'Everyone's doing their best, but the organisation's going down the pan. We're being ruined by people doing their best'.*

My fifth chemo cycle is scheduled for 10.00am. I arrive 15 minutes early – time to grab a newspaper and tea and biscuits from the ladies who sell tea and biscuits. Tea is 30p and a packet of biscuits, 20p, which seems a fair trade. I ask for ginger biscuits. Ginger biscuits, for some obscure reason are kept apart from the others – not only that, they're sold singly – 5p each. I feel as if I should lower my voice when asking for one – perhaps they're only for 'special customers', an under-the-counter product - *'nudge, nudge, wink, wink, say no more'*. I ask why they're kept apart; *'Everyone wants them'*. I hand over my 5p and feel a child-like satisfaction as I take a seat and wait my turn.

I'm called in at 10.30. I settle in; newspaper, bottle of water, sandwiches and a couple of books. The process usually takes around three hours from start to finish. I'm hooked up to the IV trolley and take a hit of glucose to begin with, before starting the two-hour chemo drip and then a 15-minute chemo drip to finish off. Only the drugs don't arrive. They're made up each morning – I have a blood test the day before and if my bone marrow count has dropped then they'll cancel the session to give it time to recover – so I can understand the 'just in time' approach. But, apparently, today, the Pharmacy has *'no staff'*. Just in time means *not* in time.

For a while nothing much happens. I read, eat my lunch (early – I'm bored) and after a couple of hours I'm given an ETA of 2.00pm. The drugs eventually turn up at 2.15. I say nothing, I'm just pleased to get started. The session finishes just after 5.00 and the pump for the 48-hour drip is connected and I'm free to go. It's been a long day. I've sat in the chair, tied to the trolley for nearly seven hours. Apart from the sheer boredom it's caused me a bag problem. I always reduce what I eat the night before so that I can get through the three-hour session beginning at 10.00am without having to empty the bag while I'm there. Although I can unplug the trolley and wheel it to the loo, emptying the bag while connected takes some dexterity. In the event I have to go – it's just been too long. I need both hands, and not being blessed with a third, I end up holding the tubes in my mouth – trying hard not to bite ...

In the end I feel there's no point in getting uptight about it and I remain sanguine – until I reach the hospital car park. As I've been parked for more than six hours I have to pay the 24-hour fee – £10. Doh!

I hit Northampton at rush hour. The road to the motorway is getting busy so I turn off and drive back to MK through the fields and villages of Northamptonshire. It's a good choice. The road undulates – in the horizontal as well as vertical plane – flanked on each side by fields of corn and stone-built villages. But for the slight reddish hue of the stonework I could be in the Cotswolds.

I arrive home to an invalid. Annie has bruised a disc in her back – through 'inappropriate' handling of a sledge-hammer (don't ask). She's in a lot of discomfort and it reminds me – as I found back in critical care in January – that no matter how bad I feel, there is always someone having a worse time than me.

We unwind sitting in the garden, salmon steaks on the BBQ. It's a lovely evening ... then I realise in the rush to leave the hospital I've not been given my steroids or anti-nausea medication. Doh! Doh!

A disease waiting to happen?

July 15th 2006

I'm reading two books at the moment – well, not simultaneously, but given the way the chemo drugs mess with my mind it would not be too difficult for Mr Grumpy to have one in one hand while Mr Happy has the other. They have both affected me in completely different ways – one for the better, the other less so.

In *Love, Medicine and Miracles* the author takes an holistic view of disease. His broad theme is that there are no incurable diseases, only incurable people. The aim, through various techniques such as meditation and visualisation, is to become an exceptional patient – one so positive that the disease can be beaten by self-healing as much as anything else. I have no problem with this at all – anything that helps is useful, although I am not good at the meditation and visualisation – I'm too impatient to relax properly. He also has the view that many doctors do not see their patients as people, but as *cases* – that becoming emotionally untangled or distant has a detrimental effect on the patient.

A key theme is the role of the mind in the progress of the disease; there is a theory that cancer is present all the time in our bodies and under normal circumstances our immune system keeps it under control. But when the immune system is unable to function properly for any reason, the cancer is able to survive and grow. He argues that our state of mind can affect the immune system in a significant way – to the extent (and I hope I'm not over simplifying his case) that cancer can be 'caused' by a poor state of mind. He says that this is not a new idea – doctors or healers, from the second century AD onwards, have observed that melancholy people are more likely to get cancer than those who are not. I can go along with the general idea. The brain controls our body in ways not completely understood, but it's highly likely that our emotions do affect our physical well-being in some way.

It's not until I read a section on the psychological profile of cancer that I become distinctly uncomfortable. At the risk again of over simplifying the good doctor, the general idea, for a male of around my age, goes something like this:

- a lack of closeness with parents, during childhood
- a difficult adolescence

- then later in life, the end of satisfying work and/or the end of a marriage.

The disease usually follows the latter events *'(for these people) within two years of the time their physiological mainstay has disappeared'.* A patient quoted in the book puts it more succinctly: *'When she walked out, the cancer walked in'.*

The idea of cancer as a disease of repressed emotion and lost self-identity is used to great effect in the poem *Miss Gee* by W.H.Auden – when the doctor in the poem comments to his wife that 'cancer's a funny thing' that attacks 'childless women' and 'men when they retire' – cancer being the outcome of their 'foiled creative fire'.

I did not have a close relationship with my parents, particularly my father. We were not a hugging family and did not show or give affection. At the time I thought nothing of it. Plenty of my friends had 'difficult' fathers – not surprising, as they'd only recently returned from the Second World War with all the horrors that that entailed. No wonder they were distant or morose or got angry easily.

My teenage years were difficult because my father was disabled and I would often have to stay home and look after him while my friends were out having fun (or making mischief). Not very cool for a Mod – complete with scooter and taste for sharp suits. This created a lot of tension and he threatened to chuck me out more than once. Again I accepted this because I realised that a lot of what was going on was to do with his frustration – he'd been an active tennis player and cricketer – and could no longer do these things. Not only that, his only son could not do these things either, try as I may. I was clumsy, inept at all sports (except riding a bike which didn't count in his view) and left school with no qualifications. My first job was digging holes for telephone poles. I was a constant disappointment to him. This is not meant to be a sob story, by the way: I'm *ex*plaining rather than *com*plaining. It's just the way it was.

He died when I was 21 – I didn't cry – I just felt an immense weight lifting from my shoulders and a sense of freedom. It would be another 20 years before I shed tears at his passing. Freed from responsibility,

I went back to school at 23, got some O levels, then a BA, a BSc and finally an MBA. I think he would have been impressed. I know I am.

By the time I got to 51 I could look back on a good(ish) career in the BBC. I had seen some amazing sights and met some amazing people. I saw it as a privilege and felt I had got as far in the organisation as I was likely to get. So when the opportunity for redundancy and early retirement came along I grabbed it with both hands. I decided not to go into freelance television production as many of my ex-colleagues did (I regarded it as a young person's game) but to use my other skills and got a part-time job with the Open University, managing projects. I'd been heavily influenced by Charles Handy (management consultant, and all-round radical thinker) – particularly when he questioned why people who act as assistants are generally younger than the people they assist. Running an organisation requires energy and enthusiasm, something that young people have in abundance. What they usually lack is wisdom and experience. So why don't people of my age sit back, let the youngsters run the show, while we throw in the occasional pearls of wisdom? This made a lot of sense to me and I was lucky enough, for a while, to work with a young enthusiastic and energetic team who appreciated my experience.

When I wasn't working at the OU I undertook a few consultancies and ran the home – cleaning, cooking and being a taxi for the children (school, dentist, doctor, etc.). It gave me a lot of satisfaction as well as an insight into the world of the part-time worker (particularly the juggling many women seem to take in their stride).

Not everyone saw my change of lifestyle in the same way I did. There were people who thought that by taking on a job with fewer responsibilities – i.e. a lower grade – I had in some way degraded myself. Sadly we still live in a society where we are measured by our job title rather than who we are. It started to get to me when I couldn't explain what I did in one word or phrase and I realised that I had lost respect in some people's eyes. At the same time my marriage started its terminal decline. I had a year of ill health ending up in hospital on two occasions, first with pleurisy and double pneumonia and then with an abscess on my appendix (hmm – a sign of things to come?).

So, these events would seem to fit the psychological profile for cancer. Where I take issue with this however, is the implication (perhaps unintended) that we can cause the disease to happen ourselves, by the way we respond to the emotional traumas in our lives. Suddenly it might be my fault. Clearly I had suppressed my feelings about my childhood and adolescence – I just accepted my lot at the time. It seemed perfectly normal. And although I had found some meaning in my post-BBC life I allowed others to undermine this. I'm not ashamed to admit that I became depressed by the culmination of events around this time. And I'm left wondering that if I had dealt with these big issues earlier I might have responded to them in a more positive way – thus possibly preventing the occurrence of the cancer.

In the event, I did sort myself out. My dog and I lived a good life – he listened patiently to all my troubles in exchange for treats and strokes. I got fit through walking him each morning, running, riding my bike and gigging with the band (and you need to be fit to sing for a couple of hours and then pack up all the gear – no roadies for the likes of us), changed my diet (to five fruit and veg a day) and ultimately found peace of mind. Then I met the wonderful Annie and so I was healthy and happy when *my* cancer walked in.

I find it hard to accept the idea that it might have been my fault. I have always put my cancer down to bad luck. Whatever mistakes I've made in my life I accept them and have few regrets. We often try to rationalise what went before – *'the past is another country'* – but unfortunately with cheap airfares these days there are regular flights there and back. For me, there is no going back. I can't go back and make it better – I can only go forwards to make it better.

I realise I'm writing intensely personal stuff here – some of the details are known only to a few close friends. And why should it be relevant to cancer? If there is a link between our emotional and our physical well-being, then it's important to understand what makes us who we are. And if we don't understand why bad things happen to us in life, we're in danger of repeating past mistakes.

The morning I read about the psychological profile for cancer I felt very low. Depression is a known side effect of chemo – there are some who advocate that depression is a side effect of cancer itself, which certainly fits in with the mind-body interaction referred to earlier. I had always assumed that because I had maintained a positive attitude to my cancer – any negative feelings only really emerging once I began chemo – that I too could become an exceptional patient. Unfortunately I didn't meet the author's strict criteria. But the author of the second book certainly did.

That morning to my great surprise and delight, the postman delivered a parcel from the USA. Some kind friends in America sent me a resource pack from the *Lance Armstrong Cancer Foundation.* Tears rolled down my cheeks as I read Lance say that we should not look on ourselves as cancer patients or cancer victims. We are all cancer *survivors* – not from the moment we get the all clear but from the moment we are *diagnosed.* It completely changed my mood and I resolved to be an exceptional patient by proxy. (So thank you Bob and Margaret).

Lance Armstrong has always been a hero of mine – not just because he won the *Tour de France* seven times or because he beat cancer – it's as much to do with *how* he beat it. I'd recommend his book, *It's Not About The Bike*, to anyone with cancer. It's not a 'how to' book – it's just the story of one man's resolve to deal with a disease which had spread in a very short time from his testicles, to his lungs and brain. His experience of chemo is harrowing – I got off lightly – but just two years later he had won the first of his seven victories. Thinking about it, I'd recommend the book to anyone – cancer or not.

I also resolved that morning to reclaim my 'creative fire'. In 1977 I was the photographer for a joint Universities expedition to Iceland. Although I took photographs after I came back, they were never as good as the ones I had taken that summer and I gradually lost interest. Now, in an attempt to simplify my life I have sold many of the toys I've accumulated over the years – recording equipment, photographic bits and pieces, computer bits, bike bits and so on. Things I no longer use or need. From now on I only keep things that are functional and attractive – a modern day William Morris I guess. I was amazed to find that the sum of my sales to date (one pair of loudspeakers and a hi-fi amp still to go if anyone's interested) allowed me to buy a Nikon Digital SLR camera. I love it and I'm all fired up to take pictures again.

In the introduction to his resource pack Lance Armstrong says the following:

'It's one thing to live, but it's another to live strong, to attack the day and attack your life with a whole new attitude. Before I had cancer I just lived, now I live strong.'

And so will I. So come on cancer – do your worst – I will beat you. Because it's not just me you're dealing with – I have friends. It's not my fault you came – you're simply an uninvited guest. Get your coat.

Little green apples

July 20th 2006

There is, on my sideboard, a fruit bowl full of green plastic apples. These polymer *pommes*, once a tacky souvenir from a French market, have come to symbolise hope – a beacon in the dark days of chemo and uncertainty. They provide a daily reminder of what I have to look forward to.

I miss fresh fruit and veggies and I sometimes worry about the effects of a diet devoid of fibre, on my long-term health. The irony of worrying about my long-term health when I have cancer is not lost on me. My cholesterol was low when I first went in to hospital – I shudder to think what it is now. Or perhaps I'll get scurvy. An unreported side effect of cancer is hypochondria, but it does have its uses.

Although it's been over six months since I've been able to eat an apple I still remember what they taste like. I fantasise about eating one. Sometimes when I'm in the supermarket I want to shove my face in the apple box, like Homer J. at the doughnut store (*hhaaarrrlll* – sound of Homer drooling). I wander around looking enviously at people putting them in their trolleys – do they know just how significant – how important – something so ordinary as an apple can be? I fear I'll end up as an apple stalker.

Malus Domestica – to give this ripened ovary of a flowering plant its proper name – has come to represent in a quite literal sense, the forbidden fruit. When all my surgery is over and the bag is finally removed – I'm guessing another nine to twelve months here – and the forbidden fruits are no longer forbidden, a crisp Granny Smith will be the first thing I eat. I don't care how small or misshapen or bruised it is – it's *numero uno* as far as I'm concerned. And it will probably be French, just like its plastic cousin.

After that it's beans on toast (wholemeal bread of course). No *Cuisine Gourmand* for me – much as I love fine food it's not what I miss. I can eat all the steak, chicken, fish even bacon sarnies (in white bread) that I want. And I do – as long as they come from happy cows, happy chickens and happy pigs. I am ignorant about the general disposition of fish, although I understand they do have a reputation as born raconteurs.[6] But it's the little guys that hide in the back of the store cupboard – the beans, pulses, chickpeas, spices – and salad stuff – that my system is craving right now.

I decided once chemo was under way that I'd have to give up eating fruit. I'd taken the risk earlier in the year of trying fruit for breakfast, just to bring some sense of normality back into my life. But anyone who has read the entry for 24th April (*Thar she blows*) will understand the devastating effect that blueberries can have on a stoma bag. The combination of fruit and chemo drugs was even more powerful – three leaks in one day. It also turns out I get no nutritional value from the fruit – fibre is processed in the large bowel which in my case, is currently resting between jobs – so everything goes straight in the bag. Apart from tasting nice it's a completely pointless exercise.

So I shall ignore the fruit counter next time I'm in the supermarket until that happy day comes when I can eat as much of the stuff as I like. But I'll keep the green plastic apples as a reminder. We've come a long way together.

[6] As in fishy stories. (I don't believe I just wrote that.)

Dear Loved Ones

July 24th 2006

'Our purpose (in life) is to help each other through this thing whatever it might turn out to be'

Kurt Vonnegut

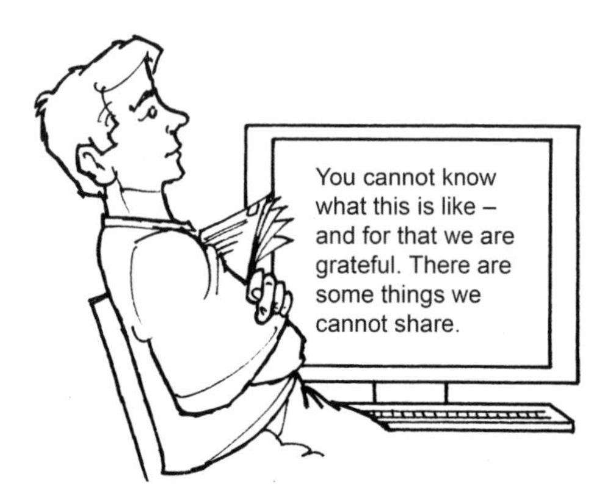

Dear Loved Ones

We know it's hard for you when you see us in pain and discomfort. You say *'I wish I could make it go away'* or *'I wish I could make it better'.* What you mean is – you wish you could make the *cause* disappear – but you can't. In that respect you're just like us – helpless. The best you can hope for is to ease the symptoms.

You cannot know what this is like – and for that we are grateful. There are some things we cannot share. Don't be hard on yourselves; if you do, we end up feeling guilty and you feel worse because you weren't able to make it better. The hardest lesson for you is to know when you can help and when you can't.

Don't forget your own needs. You are going through this as well – you need help and support. We get all the attention and it's easy for you to get left out. You may not have the disease, but you too feel pain and discomfort. So don't feel guilty about addressing your own needs. Have fun. We would in your place.

You already have an important role in our lives – you may be our partner, our parent, our sibling, our offspring, our best friend. Just carry on being that person – we won't ask any more of you.

Know that we could not do this without you. You stand on the touchline in all weathers as we play to win. You fetch our pills, you wipe our brows, you hug us when we need your warmth. You are as important to our survival as all the drugs and scans and surgery. We do know what you do for us and we love you for it. So thank you.

Yours faithfully,

Ian S.
Cancer Survivor

I am so inspired with your strong courage. A very close person of mine is diagnosed with colon cancer. Since I can't hire a nurse for her, I am doing all the messy little things. I almost give up on the bag when it leaks every day (until now actually)... When I read your diary, it made me feel that we are not alone... Someone at the other side of the world understands my situation... That's really made me relieved... Thanks... Ocean of love.

Julie
24th July 2006

This could be the last time, this could be the last time, may be the last time, I don't know

August 2nd 2006

People tell me I look well, but it's the tongue that's the giveaway. It looks, at best, like the pith of a dried, juiceless orange – at worst like a yellowed shag-pile rug – I half expect to see peanuts and cigarette butts trodden into it. This unpleasant sight, which greets me every morning in the bathroom mirror, lasts about ten days in each cycle. And then it goes, as quickly as it came.

The final two cycles have been the worst. It has had me literally on my knees, sometimes in tears, wishing it would stop. I take the anti nausea pills and go to bed and wait. Yet I know others have it far worse than me. And, it has to be said, some have it easier – although I would never argue that having chemo is easy. Perhaps my pain/discomfort threshold is simply low. I cut myself some slack when

I realise I'm dealing with three things at the same time; cancer, chemo and an ileostomy. One is enough for even the most ardent sadist.

When the pump is taken off for the last time, I ask about having the line removed – I'm keen to get this thing out of my arm. We're in tee-shirt weather now and I'm getting a little self-conscious about the stares. But they won't take it out just yet – I need a scan to see if the chemo has worked – if not I may need to go through it all again. I can't bear the thought of having more chemo. Yet I if I must, I must. I'm hoping as time passes I'll look back on this period and laugh – *'It wasn't so bad after all'* – typical British stoicism in the face of adversity: cut to scene in kitchen – family are gathered round having just received devastating news – Mother speaks; *'I'll just put the kettle on and make us all a nice cup of tea'.*

But chemo is poison; it was bad which is why I've written it down, so I don't forget. And yes, it could have been worse. My greatest fear – that I would lose my hair (while retaining my beard) and end up looking like a Morris Dancer or Narrow Boat skipper – was not realised. My bone marrow count did not drop sufficiently to cause delays in my treatment. I did not get an infection and end up hospitalised. The PICC line did not become infected. I was not stuck in bed every day. I guess the most disappointing aspect was having to cancel the charity bike ride. I simply did not have the energy to do it.

I realise that I have coped with the assault on my body. It has been far harder to cope with the assault on my mind. Depression and mood swings are par for the course, but something I had not expected was fear. Chemo is frightening because it ups the stakes – the disease is at another level now. It starts with a tumour (one if you're lucky) but soon moves from the physiological to the mathematical – it's all numbers now – stats and probabilities.

When I first went to see the liver people at Oxford they gave me a leaflet to read. I put it away, much as I did with the sample stoma bag when I was first diagnosed. Now that liver surgery is approaching I force myself to read it. I should really know better by now. These leaflets are a mix of optimism and doom. They try to be cheery, to reassure, but they can't quite pull it off because they have to give the bad news as well.

For example, only 20 years ago, one in five patients died after liver surgery – that's now around one in 20. And the liver can grow back. I guess that's a comfort. But then the sucker punch;

'Despite a successful operation, there is a risk of the cancer returning. The cancer recurs in approximately 3 out of 4 patients'.

Three out of four!!? This means on a balance of probabilities, it is more likely to return than not. I force myself to read on:

'The chances of the cancer recurring depends on the type of tumour you have'.

Ah. Now I'm confused. The leaflet does not elaborate on what is meant by different types of tumour. I'm left thinking maybe I'll be lucky, maybe I won't. Suddenly another round of chemo doesn't seem so bad if it alters the odds.

I'm trying out a new mantra; *don't count the days – make the days count*. I'd love to think this was original, but in truth I don't know if I read it somewhere and it slipped into my subconscious. Making each day count isn't as easy as it seems, but it fits in with general ethos of positive thinking, so I go along with it. I make a list of all the things I want to do – apart from beat this thing.

It turns out to be a short list – travel through Eastern Europe, Australia, Monument Valley and that's about it. That's not to say I don't have dreams – just the opposite, but it doesn't matter if I don't realise them – to me simply having dreams is part of the process; the journey we make in trying to achieve them. And the journey is as important as the destination. My ultimate dream is to expire quickly and quietly at the age of 96 having just come off stage at Glastonbury. This one dream, more than any other, sums up the importance of the journey. (Failing that, I'd like to go in my sleep like my grandfather – unlike the passengers in his car ...)

I make another list; things I've done. It's sounding a bit like count your blessings, but it's more than that – have I made the days count so far? I've been very lucky – I've found myself in some amazing places through a mix of work, holidays and just being in the right place at the right time. I've also made my own luck (recognising an opportunity when it stares me in the face – and knowing when to walk away). More than once I've been quietly minding my own business when someone says *'do you want to do X?'* and I've said *'OK'* without giving much thought to it. Sometimes what I've agreed to has terrified me but I've felt this hand pushing in my back and I've just had to go on and do it. A bit like dealing with cancer I suppose.

Here's a sample: I've seen Darwin's original specimens from the Beagle; I've ridden a horse in the Black Hills of Dakota; I've sung live on BBC (local) Radio; I've dug a tunnel under a glacier in Iceland; I've ridden a bike down a mountain in the French Alps in pitch black at the dead of night with 39 other drunks and – perhaps the most bizarre – discussed the fortunes of Charlton Athletic Football Club with three Mongolians on the Great Wall of China.

The list goes on and I think I've made the days count so far. I also realise that I don't envy anyone. Well – I sometimes wish I could play the guitar as well as Neil (from the band) but, hey, we can't all do everything. Everyone has their own list – each list is no better than any other – they are all equally valid for the people who make them. Lists are good – especially when the days are dark.

I'm already thinking beyond liver surgery – and I'm in danger of counting the days – I have a lot to look forward to next year. If the liver surgeon *'obtains clear margins'* – i.e. there's no sign of cancer beyond the tumour – then I'm home and dry. Well 'possibly' rather than 'probably'. It could always reappear at a later date somewhere else, but I'll worry about that when the time comes. It's just something every cancer survivor has to live with. The immediate issue will be dealing with surviving. I imagine many people, when they get the all clear, think *'Now what?'* What do I do next? This is where making the days count really matters. I can't go back to my old life – too much has changed. All this pain and discomfort and fear has to be for something. Saying goodbye to cancer is not enough. I have to move on – but to what?

I try and stretch the 'things to do list'. I'm not particularly adventurous or brave. I couldn't go on a death-defying ride at a fairground although I was quite happy to sit in a giant teacup at Disneyland. I've watched people hurl themselves off a mountainside attached to a parachute and, much as I'd really love to soar like a bird, I couldn't do it. I couldn't throw myself out of a plane or abseil down a cliff face as Annie has done on countless occasions. I'd be content just to hold her handbag and take photos. I really want a quiet life. And a motorbike.

I raise the topic with Annie. I fancy a Harley-Davidson *Sportster* – not a bike for leathers or going fast, but for posing around town in tee-shirt, Ray-Bans and jeans, the only concession to leather being a *fine* pair of Western boots. It is immediately obvious to me that such a bike (or rather my vision of riding it) is unsuited to the British climate – unless Global Warming gets a move on.

Annie fixes me with her teacher's look and teacher's voice (she maintains that these attributes – along with supersonic hearing and eyes in the back of the head – are standard issue for all new teachers. She even tells her class that she's allowed to keep them when she retires. Some believe her.) *'I think I'd have to put my foot down about this'.*

I think she's joking because she often uses her teacher's voice to wind me up and I make a few lame jokes about fitting stabilisers or training wheels to it. But no, the look persists and I'm suddenly transported back to over 40 years in time and I'm just about to get a detention. I've touched a nerve and the next day it all becomes clear. Dan, Annie's youngest, stops by on his way home from work. I raise the topic again. Dan, quick as a flash, pounces like Homer J. on the last pork chop: *'If Ian's having a motorbike, then I can have one.'*

I see the look – not directed at me this time – and the penny drops. It's a foolish man who comes between a lioness and her cubs.

It's a foolish man who comes between a lioness and her cubs. Or her grand cubs!!!
Even though I have seen you going through your treatments I didn't really comprehend the extent of what you have gone through so far, physically and mentally. That is until now. It has been an inspiring read and I am glad to be of your acquaintance.

Emma
12th August 2006

Halcyon days

August 14th 2006

There's a calm before the storm. Chemo is over and it's a matter of waiting to see (i) what effect it's had and (ii) when I'm likely to have liver surgery. Nothing much will happen for a while: it's like the 'phoney war', the period in 1939 after war was declared but before any significant fighting actually broke out. Like then, there are preparations to be made. I have to get fit for surgery. And not just physically, I have to prepare mentally as well. I'm not looking forward to it – no lamb to surgery this time. I know what it's like to wake up with a tube in my mouth, to surrender dignity and responsibility for bodily functions, to lose any sense of knowing what's going on.

I'm scheduled to have a CT scan and a PET scan late August/early September. They need at least six weeks for the chemo drugs to clear my system. No wonder the stuff makes you feel so bad if it hangs around that long. If it's done its job then they'll schedule a 'liver resection'.

A strange thing has happened – old yellow tongue is back. I had noted that it has a cyclical nature: it first appeared when I was having chemo, hung a round for a week or so, then disappeared leaving a healthy text-book pink tongue, only to re-emerge at the start of the next chemo session. It's been three weeks since my final dose of chemo, but it put in an appearance at the appropriate time. Not so furry as usual but yellow nevertheless and with the accompanying metallic taste in my mouth. So is this a last desperate attempt by the chemo drugs to get noticed, to let me know that they are serious players and not to be messed with or dismissed lightly? I look up 'yellow tongue' on the Internet. The consensus suggests that it's something to do with the liver. Does that mean it's a symptom of the work my liver is having to do to get rid of the chemo drugs, or is it a function of the tumour on my liver? I guess only time will tell.

I've been needing a nap in the afternoon because the chemo has been so fatiguing, but I'm now getting through most days without one. It depends what I've been doing in the day, but it's progress. I have to go the hospital once a week to have the line flushed, and I resolve to go by bike next time rather than drive.

I've been trying to do some decorating but don't have the energy right now, so I'm back to sitting in the garden, with a pair of binoculars watching Annie paint the living room ceiling – the binoculars are useful to see if she's missed a bit.

I risk forbidden fruits as normality slowly returns – a glass of champagne (grapes) to celebrate Annie's mother's 80th birthday and sticky toffee pudding (containing dried fruit) at a lunch to celebrate the birthday of Annie's eldest son, Chris. A friend of Annie's declares that sticky toffee pudding is better than sex. While I agree that sticky toffee pudding is indeed one of the finest desserts to be had, I really think he ought to get out more.

I have just read your comments and have cried at your enthusiastic outlook and sheer determination at such a difficult time in your life. I am 33 years old and have recently been told that I need to have a permanent colostomy as a result of childbirth. I do not have cancer. I have been feeling sorry for myself lately, and have been struggling to deal with the idea of living with this bag attached to me. Having read your comments, I felt the need to write. You are an inspiration to all cancer sufferers. I am going to enjoy every day of my life (bag or no bag) and enjoy my four children. I am going to live strong every day. I am going to stop complaining about silly things and have a positive attitude. I wish you well and will keep you in my prayers

Trish

17th August 2006

The cost of living (with cancer)

August 21st 2006

The Halcyon days are over and a storm breaks. It's not the storm I was expecting however. I've now been off work for more than 28 weeks so my entitlement to Statutory Sick Pay from my employer has ended. This means my salary will drop by around £300 per month. To make up the deficit I'm advised by my employer to claim Incapacity Benefit – which neatly works out at around £300 per month. This is something I did not anticipate having to do back in January.

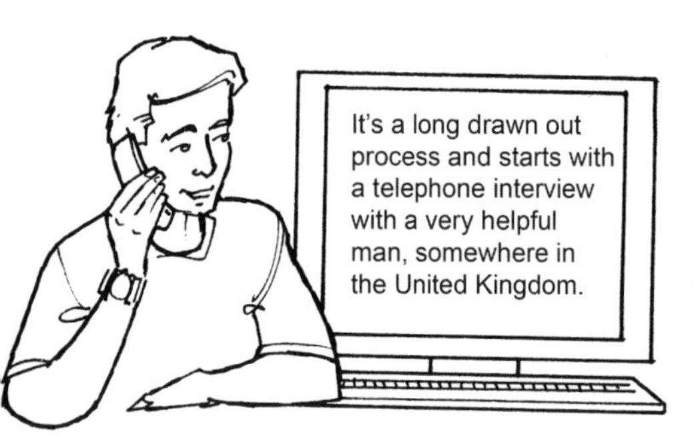

It's a long drawn out process and starts with a telephone interview with a very helpful man, somewhere in the United Kingdom. He explains that this benefit is not means tested and as I'm already in work, my claim will be straightforward. What follows is anything but straightforward.

Shortly afterwards I get a letter summarising the interview. The envelope has a Belfast postmark. Next I get a phone call from the local Job Centre in Bletchley. They want proof of my identity and ask if I can bring my passport in. I explain that I cannot do this right away as I'm having a bad time with the chemo. That's alright they say – someone can bring it in for you. So Annie goes off to the Job Centre with my passport. I'm now wondering if I am missing something; someone who is clearly not me – wrong gender, wrong name – is showing them my passport to prove my identity. I assume it's the drugs messing with my mind and that this is all perfectly normal.

Two weeks later I get a letter bearing a Portsmouth postmark asking for a medical certificate from my GP. Now I'm really confused. I start to wander off into the realms of fantasy (these drugs are strong) – could all these communications come from the same person wandering around the UK? The speed of communication suggests they may be travelling by bicycle. Or perhaps they have an auntie in

Portsmouth. Maybe she was visiting at the time, and they asked her to post the letter and she didn't remember until she arrived back home. I feel I'm in the middle of a Kafka novel. Or perhaps I'm just barking mad.

I start to look forward to the next communication. I consider putting a map of the UK on the wall and sticking little flags in the towns and cities to coincide with the postmarks and phone calls. I soon dismiss the idea realising that I must be a really sad person if my idea of excitement is plotting the trail of letters from the Department of Work and Pensions. Still – I do wonder where the next one will come from ...

I write back to the person in Portsmouth explaining that I have already sent in a letter from my consultant saying that I will not be fit to return to work for the remainder of 2006. This is not good enough and I have to get a note from my GP. I protest that my GP is busy and will not know the details of my case as well as the consultant. Deaf ears. I duly go to my local surgery and get signed off for a month.

It's obvious that I do not understand the system. I have not been out of work since the age of 16. Even when I went to university in my late 20s I took unpaid leave from my then employer, continued to pay National Insurance and so have a continuous employment record stretching back 43 years. Which means I have never claimed anything from the State before, so it's all new to me. The paperwork is confusing and although the people are helpful, the phone lines always seem to be engaged. Everybody's doing their best ...

... Or are they? My good humour is tested by another letter from Portsmouth. My claim for Incapacity Benefit has been turned down – because I have a pension from my previous employer. What?? Incapacity Benefit is *not* means tested. But if they take my pension into account then surely it is? Or am I missing something again? I gave them details of my income over a month ago. Why wait until now to tell me?

The drop in income is a big deal right now. Cancer is an expensive business – I have to travel to hospitals in Northampton and Oxford as well as MK; hospital car park fees can reach hundreds of pounds over a year; my diet is now more expensive than it was – and to accommodate this fatty, protein-laden diet I have to add in the cost of BIG trousers. I'm also paying people to do things I cannot manage to do myself. It all adds up.

I check the Dept of W&P website – and sure enough, if you scroll down far enough it mentions pensions. But no explanation as to why people with pensions are means tested. It's not just about me anymore – there must be many people in a similar situation – drawing an occupational pension while taking on part-time work to supplement income. And this number will surely rise as the population ages. Current figures show that the majority of people will not have sufficient pension to manage on. So working and drawing a pension will become a necessity for many. I resolve to write to my MP about it. In the meantime I realise I'm going to have to go back to work while I wait for the next stage in my treatment. I phone the Occupational Health unit at work to make an appointment with their doctor to see if they'll let me come back for a while.

Then to rub salt into the wound, another letter from Belfast – this time stating that my Incapacity Benefit will be subject to Income Tax. How? – when I'm not getting it? After two days of the busy tone I finally speak to a very helpful young man in the Portsmouth office. I ask him the following;

Mr Grumpy: *'If I earned £100,000 per year and had £100,000 in savings could I claim Incapacity Benefit?'*
Helpful Young Man: *'Yes'*

Mr Even-More Grumpy: *'Are you sure?'*
Helpful Young Man: *'Yes.'*

Mr E-M G: *'Why?'*
HYM: *'Incapacity Benefit is not means tested.'*

He cannot (*HE cannot??!!*) understand why those with a pension should have it taken into account. He thinks it wrong and unfair. He offers to get the person who made the decision to phone me and explain, as he can't. In the meantime a news item on the BBC[7] states that the Dept of W&P has paid out £13,000,000 in benefits over the past three years to people in prison – even though they're not entitled to any. And now I'm sounding like someone who writes letters to the newspapers complaining about 'benefit scroungers'. Which I'm not. I simply cannot understand how something which is not meant to be means-tested clearly is.

I feel as strongly about this issue as I do about the NHS illegally forcing people to sell their homes in order to pay for long-term healthcare[8]. Not that I think people in the NHS are crooks – I'm sure they're doing their best to meet Government financial targets, but may be misinterpreting the rules in order to save money – at the expense of those entitled to that money. And in spite of numerous court cases they continue to do it.

This all confirms a long-held belief that middle-income people of my generation (the baby boomers) will end up paying for healthcare, in one way or another, as we get older. Annie and I are not wealthy – neither are we poor. Apart from the financial black-hole known as children, we are, like many people, comfortable in that we don't have debts other than a mortgage and we have some savings. The State will, quite rightly, continue to look after the needy and the wealthy can afford to look after themselves.

So, if you fall into the middle-income group and are planning on having a life-threatening disease sometime in the future, do consult a financial advisor first and put together a plan that will leave you either very poor or very wealthy. Whatever you do, don't stay in the middle. Or have a pension and work.

If, at the end of the day I don't get Incapacity Benefit, I'll accept the decision – as long as I can understand it. If not, I'll continue to fight – for others as well as myself. Cancer survivors have enough to deal with without worrying about money. I know it's all relative – I'm not homeless, I don't go hungry and I can pay my way. And I only have one tumour on my liver – I met a man in chemo who had four. I guess it's become a matter of principle, and it diverts my attention from thinking about the next stage in my treatment.

I realise it's the cancer that's made me bolshie. I'm usually quite compliant in the face of authority. Annie notices I've got really angry over the past few months. Every single day I think about life and death. Not in a morbid way – I simply confront my demons – get them out and have a good hard look at them, so I know what I'm dealing with. A news item on the BBC News[9] website today: those with advanced bowel cancer living in Wales are refused a new cancer drug. It's not deemed cost-effective even though it's widely used in Europe. Then the sting – *'The five year survival rate for patients with advanced bowel cancer is less than 5%'.* This is why I have to confront my demons – I'm determined to be one of the 5% – but first I have to get a scan. I ring Oxford, there are 300 people waiting for scans, I'm somewhere on the list. Ring back in three days to find out just where.

Sometimes I have to fight really hard to remain positive, so I guess the frustration just spills over into other areas. I'm trying to learn how to assert my rights without being rude or aggressive. After two days, I'm still waiting for that phone call from the Dept of W&P. Perhaps they're off on their bike again. I call this morning and speak to someone else who admits Incapacity Benefit *is* means tested for two groups of people – those with private health insurance (fair enough) and those with a pension. He also says it's unfair, he doesn't understand the reason either – *'We don't make the rules – it's the Government'.* He then bends my ear about how unfair Inheritance Tax is. As a parting shot he suggests trying to claim for a 'disability living allowance' – *'It might help but they're slower than us'.*

OK, so I'm not going to win this one, but I will write to my MP. Like I said, it's become a matter of principle.

And now a joke about the cost of healthcare, just to prove that my encounter with the Department of Work and Pensions has not left me bitter and twisted (and apologies if you've heard it before).

A woman brought a very limp Cocker Spaniel to the veterinary surgery. As she laid her pet on the table, the vet pulled out his stethoscope and listened to the dog's chest. After a moment or two, the vet shook his head sadly and said, *'I'm so sorry, your pet has passed away'.*

The distressed owner wailed, *'Are you sure?'*
'Yes, I'm sure. The dog is dead,' he replied.

'How can you be so sure?' she protested. *'I mean, you haven't done any testing on him or anything. He might just be in a coma or something.'*

The vet rolled his eyes, turned around and left the room. He returned a few moments later with a black Labrador retriever. As the dog's owner looked on in amazement, the Labrador stood on his hind legs, put his front paws on the examination table and sniffed the dead Cocker from top to bottom. He then looked at the vet with sad eyes and shook his head.

The vet petted the Labrador retriever, took him out of the room, and returned a few moments later with a beautiful cat. The cat jumped up on the table and also sniffed the limp Cocker from head to tail and back again. The cat sat back on its haunches, shook his head, meowed softly, jumped down and strolled out of the room.

The vet looked at the woman and said, *'I'm sorry, but as I said, your dog is most definitely, 100% certifiably, dead'.*

Then the vet turned to his computer terminal, hit a few keys, and produced a bill, which he handed to the woman. The dog's owner, still in shock, took the bill. *'£250!'* she cried. *'£250 just to tell me my dog is dead?'*

The vet shrugged. *'I'm sorry. If you'd taken my word for it, the bill would have been £20. But with the Lab Report and the Cat scan, it all adds up.'*

I have just discovered your blog Ian. I work within the hospice system on a voluntary basis. Eight weeks ago my younger sister was diagnosed with bowel cancer and despite being close she has refused to allow me to visit her during her six week period of chemo and radio therapy. We keep in touch by texting and I send her cards, etc. I just want to say just how much your entry 'Dear Loved Ones' has helped me this morning. I am standing with my arms open wide waiting for the moment when I can see my sister again, when she is ready. Your site is an inspiration and your sense of humour is beyond price. Bless you.

Barbara
24th August 2006

Hi Ian, Just keep hitting that DWP wall is all I can say!
I went through similar, but not an interview. Details of my IB entitlement were sent to a 10+ yr old address – that the DWP had separately wrote and asked me for, although the original form said I didn't need to provide previous addresses unless I had been living at my present address for less than three years (I hadn't)!!
Then, having been advised of the IB payment (via the tax deduction letter you refer to) I was due, for some reason one month of payment was missed. After the usual phone calls (and engaged tones), I was told they didn't know why this had happened but would sort it out. Another two months later, and guess what – yep, another missed payment. My advice? Watch your bank account details and check that you're paid when they say you will be.

All the best for the future, Kim.
26th August 2006

[7] BBC News online (http://news.bbc.co.uk/1/hi/uk_politics/5262890.stm) *Inmates receive benefits millions:* August 18th 2006.
[8] *The National Homes Swindle: a growing scandal*; Panorama, BBC1 July 23rd 2006.
[9] BBC News online (Health) August 26th 2006.

Liver and bacon

August 25th 2006

A letter arrives from the John Radcliffe Hospital, Oxford. I'm to be admitted for the liver operation on the 2nd October. I'm a little surprised and somewhat elated. I park my fears about the operation to one side for now. I'm surprised because I've not yet managed to get any scans booked and elated because I feel things are moving again after months of chemo, which seemed like a lot of pain and discomfort for no apparent gain. I get on the phone to Oxford and although there's a long waiting list I get a CT scan in two weeks' time. The PET scan is arranged for next week. Result.

My initial reaction to the October date is shared, to some extent, by Annie. She's relieved that things are moving on, but I can tell she's apprehensive. Oxford is 50 miles away and visiting will be difficult. Once she's locked in her classroom, she may as well be on the dark side of the moon. She's also read the same literature about liver surgery as I have. Each time I've felt bad and scared she's been there for me — so positive and supportive. She's put her own fears to one side for my sake. Now it's my turn to support her — so it's good that I'm feeling upbeat about it all. I am assuming, of course, that the scans prove positive.

I felt like this in January just after I got the date for the bowel operation; I know the fears will return the nearer I get to October. In the meantime I have five weeks to prepare. And if all it goes according to plan, I'll be home in about ten days *sans* tumour. I celebrate the news with a cup of freshly brewed coffee and a bacon roll. Bliss. It's the simple things in life that give the greatest pleasure and are so often overlooked.

Annie's been painting the sitting room and apart from offering tea and encouragement, I've made some legs for a TV unit we've rescued. Well, when I say legs, I mean blocks of wood. But it means getting to grips with a plane. And that's another simple pleasure — shaping wood with a carpenter's plane. I love wood; the colour, smell and feel of it. I'm using mahogany for this project — I have a wood store full of odds and ends (I hate to throw wood away) — it always comes in useful. Peter Kay once said that you can tell when you're turning into your dad when you keep a piece of wood just for stirring paint.

I guess it's why I like guitars so much. The idea that a piece of wood and some steel strings can look and sound so beautiful never ceases to amaze me. I'd have a house full of them if I had room (and the money).

These legs/blocks are tapered which means planing at an angle of around 30° to the horizontal. School woodwork classes often required me to plane horizontally which I never managed to do successfully — now I have to plane at an angle, my school experience comes in handy.

The chemo drugs are gradually leaving my body. It's not a fond farewell: I'm glad to see the back of them. Most of the side effects have gone — I still get some bleeding from the stoma and I'm managing to get through the day without a nap – but I'm exhausted by evening. Sometimes, if I'm tired during the day, I force myself to carry on; I need to get stronger. The band has seven gigs between now and October. I cancel one in Leicester as it's nearly a full day's work with three hours travelling, then a good four hours setting up, performing and packing up. I just can't do it right now. But I will in time.

Annie's eldest son, Chris, came over to help me lay a new floor in the sitting room. In truth, I helped him. It was an absolute pleasure – he's a hard-working lad – and we devised a system for working together and just got on with it. I struggled to keep up with him, but I was so pleased at the end of the day to have a nice new maple floor and to have managed a degree of physical labour. I'm exhausted – every bone in my body aches – but I have a sense of normality that I've not experienced for months. It reinforces my determination not to give in to this disease or its fallout and I now have a new mantra – *'I'm going to beat cancer if it kills me'.*

Zen and the art of stoma maintenance (or how I learned to stop worrying and love the bag)

August 29th 2006

'Adjusting to life with a stoma takes courage at first, because it requires some practical skills and planning.'

http://www.fittleworth.net

It's taken me about six months to get to the stage where I can change the bag in under three minutes. I don't think I'll ever be totally at ease with it, but I am managing to deal with most of what it chucks at me. Which is quite a lot sometimes.

I've developed a routine, which seems to work most of the time and I've learned not to panic when things go wrong. And I have also learned there is far more to stomas and bags than meets the eye.

Know your stoma

An ostomy is a generic term for a surgically created opening where the inside of the body is exposed to the outside world (a bit like hanging, drawing and quartering, only without the hanging or quartering). The most common are probably colostomy (involving the large bowel) and ileostomy (involving the small bowel). A stoma is what actually emerges from the body.

I have a loop ileostomy – a loop of the small bowel (the ileum) protrudes from an opening in the right-hand side of my stomach. It's a bit like a bicycle inner tube, folded back on itself and then poked through a hole. It has a puncture – a small hole in the sticky-out-bit allows waste material to flow into the bag. A loop ileostomy is designed to be a temporary diversion – when all my cancer surgery is finished, the puncture will be repaired and the tube pushed back from whence it came (or at least that's the theory).

There's no getting away from it – a stoma is a pretty weird thing. As soon as I eat anything, an impulse starts my insides working. The stoma moves in concert with the passage of food down my gullet. Nothing may actually emerge – it just likes to be involved. I guess it has a bit of an ego (it's all me, me, me with stomas) because it also starts moving when I sing. This impulse (the food bit at least) happens to all of us – I only know about it because it's on the surface and can see and feel it. Otherwise I'd have no idea what was going on. And it doesn't stop at the stoma. Sometimes I feel a desperate need to open my bowels – the sensation has been so real that I've rushed to the loo – but nothing emerges. Except on two occasions, when I've discharged clear mucus. It's very disconcerting when it happens and worried me at first. It's known in the trade as a 'phantom poo' (I'm not making this up). I assume this means my large colon is still working, despite the trauma of surgery.

The ideal output is meant to have the consistency of porridge (ironic as I can't eat it). I've seen medical staff get positively excited about the contents of my bag – it reminds me of Goldilocks and the Three Bears – *'This porridge is too runny, this porridge is too stodgy, but this porridge is just right'.*

My porridge was not the same when I was undergoing chemotherapy. The drugs mess with the digestive system and sometimes it was like Branston pickle (sorry – I guess Boxing Day will never be the same again) and at others, like a badly poured pint of Brown Ale (too much head). I had other drugs to change the output, but decided not to bother – I was already taking too many drugs and decided to live with the inconvenience.

A stoma can be incredibly noisy. Mine gurgles, splutters – even whistles on occasion (but not any recognisable tune though). I was embarrassed at first when it kicked off while other people were around – especially those who didn't know I had a bag. They would look puzzled – knowing roughly what the sound was, but not knowing where it was coming from. After a while I stopped being embarrassed – life's just too short.

It was very fashionable a few years ago to wear the stoma long. It would hang two to three inches from the surface of the stomach, like some sort of proboscis. But times change and now short is all the rage. It's worth mentioning that patients do not get a choice about stoma length – that's a surgeon thing. The advantage of a long stoma is that the contents of the bowel are delivered safely into the bag. The disadvantage is that it looks pretty hideous. Short may be stylish but short means the bag is more likely to leak. The occurrence of leaking bags appears to have risen as stomas have shrunk (I bet there's a PhD there). A leaking bag is one of the most upsetting, depressing, irritating, messy and, frankly, unnecessary aspects of living with a stoma. My record was three leaks in one day, but I've just had an email from someone who beat that with four in one day. Getting a bag that works is vital.

Know your bag

I woke up in intensive care with a bag in place. Apart from a few days before Christmas when I was given a present of bag samples by the Bag Lady, it was the first time I'd seen one (I binned them as soon as I got home – I just couldn't face it). Just to confuse matters it had been fitted upside down – I heard one of the nurses remark *'what are we supposed to do – turn him upside down to empty it?'* As far as I was concerned a bag was a bag. It was nothing to do with me. It took another three weeks before I could look at it. It leaked frequently – I would have to ask someone to empty it and if they were busy it could take hours. The day I took responsibility for emptying it myself (a condition of coming home) was a milestone in my recovery.

I assumed that all bags were alike – any differences I'd noticed were purely cosmetic as far as I was concerned. I also assumed that the leaks were down to me either not attaching the bag properly or because of my diet. It simply didn't occur to me that leaks could be a function of stoma design or bag design.

There are two fundamental elements to bag design: the way it opens (for emptying) and the way it attaches to the body. The latter is the more significant.

The back of most bags – the sticky part that attaches to the stomach – has a flat profile. This is the sort I used for the first few months. It leaked every few days; sometimes due to my poor technique, sometimes because I was eating too much fruit for it to handle – fruit goes through the system like an express train – and also because as I regained weight the shape of my stomach changed, meaning that it became a poor fit. Even the hairs on my stomach, as they grew back after surgery, caused problems, acting as a conduit to the outside world for runny porridge desperate to escape.

A poorly fitting bag not only causes leaks, it damages the skin around the stoma. When I took the bag off to change it I would be confronted by a mess, not only from the 'porridge', but also by raw skin (think nappy rash). For a long time I assumed that this was normal. It all came to a head when I began chemo and the bag leaked three times in one morning. My Bag Lady suggested a different design of bag.

My current bag has a convex profile. This means it pushes into my stomach, thereby forcing the stoma to protrude more than it would do otherwise. The adhesive pad is also thicker than standard, and just to make sure, it comes with a belt (I thought about getting matching gloves and a scarf, but that's probably a bit OTT). It's a little uncomfortable but I've had no leaks since May. When I change the bag there is no mess – my stoma now looks like the ones in the stoma care leaflets. So why aren't all bags like this? The convex design has one major flaw. If it pushes in too far (i.e. the profile is too convex) it can cause the stoma to prolapse and it'll not just be porridge that ends up in the bag, but the stoma itself. And we wouldn't want that, would we?

So all bags are a compromise. This particular one works for me. But there is a bewildering array of bags out there – just look on any manufacturer's or supplier's website (eg. Fittleworth Medical). So how do you choose the right one? Or ensure that it continues to work properly? This is where the Bag Lady comes in. I see her every three weeks or so for a service. She even shaves around the stoma and gives it the full beauty treatment. Get to know your Bag Lady/Man. I am lucky to have a Bag Lady who is also an angel.

Know yourself

Living with a stoma takes confidence. As I've said before I shy away from the courage bit because courage/bravery implies choice. If Annie were to change my bag then she would truly be courageous, because she doesn't have to do it. But I do – I have no choice – therefore I am not courageous. I was/still am squeamish to some extent, although that has changed a little over the past few months.

I do go along with the other advice on the Fittleworth website though; it does help to plan. I now have a routine, which I try to stick to. I change the bag after I've showered, usually in the mornings, when the stoma is quiet. I then arrange all the paraphernalia – pink disposable bag, wipes, kitchen roll, new bag (already cut out to fit), adhesive remover and a plastic bag for rubbish – on a bathroom stool.

Although the bag is waterproof, the shower tends to loosen the adhesive around the top. And although I can now change the bag quickly I don't rush the process – I allow about half an hour – so that the area around the stoma is thoroughly dry – the new bag won't stick if it's wet. I think the taking time part is vital. In the early days, particularly when a bag had leaked, I would rush to put a new one on only to find that it too would leak, my haste causing new problems.

My routine does not always work though. Sometimes if I'm in a hurry I take chances – like I did this morning. I was late for an appointment and could see that the stoma was slightly active. This has happened before and I've been so confident that I've removed the bag without worrying about it – knowing that I could catch any discharge. But this morning the stoma erupted with an intensity I'd not seen for ages – down my groin and legs – and all over the new bag that I was just about to attach. I sat there stemming the flow with some kitchen roll wondering what to do next. I had no new bags to hand, so I was stuck. In the end Annie found a new box of bags and I sorted myself out. It doesn't pay to be over-confident.

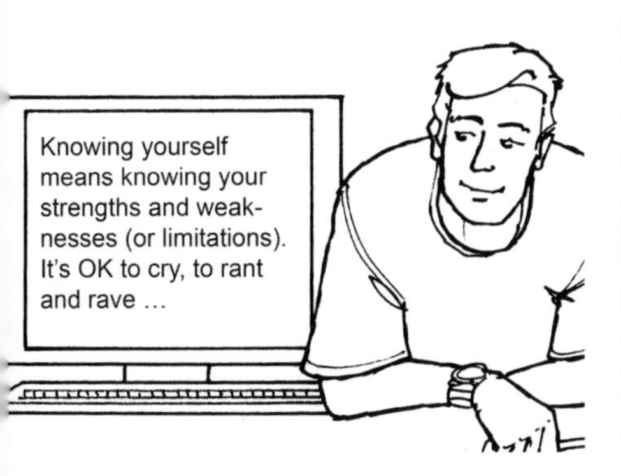

Knowing yourself means knowing your strengths and weaknesses (or limitations). It's OK to cry, to rant and rave, to feel it's *sooo* unfair. That's normal. A stiff upper lip is not a particularly attractive feature and is highly over-rated. And we're each allowed to have our own ways of dealing with it (just as long as we don't hurt other people). I'm never angry or depressed because I have cancer – that's just bad luck. But I do sometimes get angry and depressed by the consequences.

It's taken me a long time to recognise my strengths. But I've got there. And I know my limitations – I'm reluctant to travel too far from home (or a disabled loo). Dealing with the bag while out can be a pain. Few pubs have disabled loos – try sitting sideways to empty the bag in a cubicle – and so I've had to turn down gigs and invitations that have involved travelling. I know some people with ileostomies go on holidays, but I'm not ready to risk it: my worst nightmare is trying to deal with the bag in an aircraft loo. I'm not embarrassed about this – I know a time will come when this will change. But not right now. I'm confident that I'm dealing with the bag in the best way I can for now. My district nurse often uses a Jamaican phrase when I ask how he is

– *'I'm just taking a rough life easy'* – and that sums up stoma care up for me. Living with a stoma is rough. So take it easy.

You are an inspiration. I am hoping that my sister will feel like seeing me in a couple of weeks. One word and I'll be on the A24 like a rocket !! I am making this journey with her and I too have lessons to learn. We shall carry the 2nd October in our minds and hearts for you. Just keep on making music – there is nothing like it.

Barbara
29th August 2006

Hello Ian, my name is John and after reading about your website in the Cancer Research UK magazine I thought that you might like to know that I have been through a similar experience to you. I was diagnosed with bowel cancer in early December 2005 and within a week I had had a scan and was admitted to hospital for the operation. I had an ileostomy straight away, unlike you, and made a quick recovery so they let me home on Christmas Eve so I was able to spend Christmas Day with friends and family. I started chemo about four weeks later but, unfortunately, after about six days I had such a bad reaction to it, that I ended up back in hospital on a drip for eight days with a badly ulcerated mouth and tongue so they took me off chemo immediately. I also had trouble with bag leaks until the Stoma Nurse put me on convex bags. I suppose the flat bags must be cheaper so they try them first. After a while I did have a prolapse of the stoma so in April 2006 I had the ileostomy reversed. At first I wondered if I had done the right thing as I was in and out of the toilet all day long so I phoned up to see if everything was all right to be told that it was normal and that things would improve as weeks went by. This has proved to be the case and I am now back to something approaching normality. Recently, I have had another scan and a colonoscopy and the results have been negative so in spite of the fact that I missed out on the chemo, everything seems to be alright. I hope that this e-mail has been some help to you when it comes to making a choice about whether to have your own ileostomy reversed.

Best wishes, John
30th August 2006

I had bowel cancer in 1996. I was diagnosed in May, had radiotherapy in June and July, was operated on in September, had the 'bag' reversal in December, and had chemotherapy for about 20 weeks after that. Like you Ian I had 'fun' with the bag, the loop had a mind of its own at times, and I had a few tantrums because of it. I have now been clear for 10 years and lead a normal life but have to be careful about certain items of food which can create potentially embarrasing situations (French onion soup) springs to mind! My purpose in writing this Ian is to keep on with your positive attitude and to wish you the very best of luck and hope that like so many bowel cancer sufferers you make a full recovery soon.

Best Wishes, Ralph
1st September 2006

Look at me – I'm dancing

September 3rd 2006

'Pain is temporary, quitting is forever.'

Lance Armstrong

He's right of course. Even now I can't really remember what it felt like in January, February or March. Chemo is still fresh in my mind, but it is fading fast. So as I approach liver surgery I should try and remember that the pain and discomfort will go. It's not really that that bothers me – it's the operation itself. Although the success rate has improved dramatically over the past 20 years or so, it's still scary. The liver consultant tells me that the first three days are critical. If I get through that with no or few complications then I should be home and dry (unlike the bowel op where complications tend to arise after the first three days).

I also have to remember that under X-ray my liver does not look like a Dalmatian: I have one spot, not 101. So the stats for liver surgery need to be placed in context. I resolve not to read any more news items about bowel cancer – without any explanation of the extent of the disease it just scares the pants off me. I have a PET scan and a CT scan next week and a meeting with the consultant to discuss the results on the eighth. If the chemo's done its job, I assume I'll get the green light for the op in October.

Having just read Lance Armstrong's second book[10], I look longingly at my bikes. I must get a couple of rides in: it's now only four weeks or so until surgery – where does the time go? I cycle to the hospital for a line flush and to have the dressings changed. It's not far but there are a couple of hills *en route* (OK, mole hills, but to me they could be the Alps) and I'm puffed when I get there. I'm also puffed when I get back. But I'm glad I did it. I would like to go out on my racing bike with its cool new carbon fibre forks before the end of the month, but need to work up to it. I'm also a little nervous about Lycra shorts and the bag; not a pretty sight. I wonder about a bag in carbon fibre.

I'm also going back to work for a couple of weeks. I'm a bit nervous about that too. I'll have been off for eight months; things have changed a lot in that time, people have come and gone and I'll be like the new boy at school again. I've noticed that when you first join an organisation, you don't know anyone; then after a while you do get to know everyone, then after you've been there too long, you don't know anyone again.

The band had a gig on Saturday; an outdoor music festival sort of thing. As it was in the open air and September, it rained and howled. It did not dampen my spirits though. We sat around in the pub before going on stage, laughing and telling jokes and Tim (the bass player) remarked that it was just like old times. In other words I seemed 'normal' – back to my old self from the period BC (before cancer). It is such a strange time – I do feel normal, I'm getting my strength back and apart from the bag, the line in my arm and this thing on my liver, I look much like anyone else.

We're a sort of Tex-Mex band (accordion, mandolin, guitars and upright bass) in terms of arrangements and our songs (from the 30s to the noughties) are full of Latin-American rhythms and riffs, with a bit of Blue-Grass, Old-Time and Reggae thrown in, which means a lot of toe-tapping. As the singer I get to step back from the mike a lot of the time while the band play instrumental breaks. I cannot keep still and end up dancing around on stage. I was lost in one particular tune and suddenly looked up at the wind-blown and rain-soaked crowd; I wanted to shout out '*Look at me, I've got cancer and I'm dancing*', not to show off, but simply to say, '*I'm normal*'. But I didn't. I thought it might scare them off or darken the mood, which is the last thing I wanted.

Some of our regular fans (we do have them) have followed my progress through the band's website and it is always good to get their support and encouragement, especially when I forget the words or arrangements, as I have done on occasion. I blame the drugs. One thing that cancer has taught me is not to underestimate people's ability to care.

By chance my ex-sister-in-law (or sister as I now prefer to call her) is the same blood group as me – B Rhesus positive. Not exactly hen's teeth, but not plonk. She offers to bank a couple of pints for me just in case – blood transfusions are not uncommon during liver resections. This is an amazing offer, but I decline. As Anthony Aloysius St John Hancock once said *'That's very nearly an armful'.*

I am constantly amazed by people, not only those close to me, but also those I don't know – *'the kindness of strangers'*. I've had a steady trickle of comments to my blog, but since it featured in the August edition of the Cancer Research UK newsletter, the trickle has increased. Some who write have been through it, others are carers or supporters. Some take from what I've written, others give, but all offer encouragement. So thank you all who've emailed or left comments, it's much appreciated.

No matter how tough it gets, I realise there is a cancer community out there, willing to offer support. In the words of Sister Sledge *'We are Family'*. We are not alone.

Hi Ian! I really wish you well for your operation next month, 'only' one spot on your liver – great news as far as it goes from what I know about this disease. I say that because my Dad has the same cancer as yourself, bowel, jumped to his liver, had a resection and that part of his liver is all clear now and functioning perfectly – well enough to digest his red wine anyways!!!! He has 10–11 spots on the other side but his surgeons said if they operated they could kill him in case they nick 'something' and it spreads it. Dad has one in his cisterna chyli behind his liver – part of the lymph system but still bowel cancer, not lymphatic I might add. He and Mum are off to Canada soon for a well deserved break!!! He has had this now for two years this month, he'll probably be back on chemo Nov/Dec after his CT scan. As long as it keeps working and 'knocking' them back, as we all say, then that is all we may hope and pray for. If the chemo doesn't work too well this time, God willing another one will – a new one. I have a dreadful fear that I might lose Dad but, like yourself, he is sooooo fit and looks absolutely bloody normal – sometimes we joke that there must have been a mix up at the hospital with records or something! What I am trying to say is that your words give me hope for Dad, I cannot talk much about it with him as I cry every time. My mum was my age now, about 35, when she lost her mum to cancer and that puts the fear of God into me. You are in extremely capable hands and your treatment is working, your operation will be a complete success and I expect you'll be a lucky person in a few years to be told that you are in remission. Yours has probably been 'caught' in the nick of time and like Dad your general healthy lifestyle will help you beat this thing and keep going on to live a normal life. I am sorry if I babble too much but this is obviously something close to my heart too and I can imagine what your family is going through. I won't say that I can imagine what you're going through as only you can. Keep positive and it'll be OK. xxx.xxx.

Cath

5th September 2006

Hi Ian I am one of the, no-doubt, many who will see your article in the Cancer Research newsletter. I was diagnosed at 36 with breast cancer almost five years ago (still too scary to call it five years as it's not until October, the 30th actually). Reading your diary reminded me of the journal I kept during a counselling course I recently finished – it gave me somewhere to spill it out and explore my thoughts. I am glad you have found it helpful and hopefully others will too. I also hope that it helps people to talk about things and not turn their faces away from our realities. Some of the things you have said have particularly resonated within me – I read about your bag issues and was reminded of my own with my prosthesis. Very different I know – my attachment is made to be seen and yours to be disguised. It took me a very long time to get anywhere being OK about it, or my wigs. The other resonance was from your mention of normality. Seeing as you seem to like quotes, I am a fan of Terry Pratchett who described alternative universes as being like going down the wrong trouser leg. Every so often I find myself aware of which leg I am in – CancerWorld or NormalWorld ... and it's so surreal being in CancerWorld and surrounded by beings in NormalWorld.
Take care, and all the best for the op.

JJ
5th September 2006

Thanks for this JJ.
I like your description of Cancerworld and Normalworld. Maybe in time it gets easier to move between the two?
As for my bag being disguised – I'm thinking of cashing in my Scottish ancestry and getting a kilt – that way I could wear the bag on the outside (i.e. sporran) which would be a lot more convenient.
Take care and thanks for writing.

Ian
6th September 2006

[10] *Every Second Counts*; Lance Armstrong, (Yellow Jersey Press, 2004).

The working life

September 8th 2006

The first thing that surprised me was the computer. After spending the last eight months or so at home using a Mac, the old office PC was a bit of a shock. Not just the clunky keyboard and mouse, but also the software. I've been spoilt.

The second thing was the price of coffee in the canteen – 75p. I could get a fish supper, a ride home on the bus and still have change ... I really have been spoilt.

The third thing was a (half full/half empty – depending on your point of view) jar of coffee and a packet of biscuits on my bookshelf, sitting there since before last Christmas. At least I washed my cup before I went off on sick leave – unlike a colleague who, on returning from a summer break found a long, grey, hairy growth clinging to the side of her coffee pot and it was not the new Head of Department.

People were pleased – and surprised – to see me. It was a nice welcome back. As I wandered over to the canteen I got to see the campus with fresh eyes. I am lucky to work in an environment where my office is surrounded by mature trees and green fields. The trees in particular are magnificent – an ancient mulberry tree, a couple of cedars of Lebanon and a huge copper beech. There are also fruiting shrubs and trees and although it's sunny, there is a hint in the air of a change of season, confirmed by the elderberries, blackberries and crab apples. As I take in these sights I half expect to hear Beethoven's 6th blaring out from the greenery.

The only thing to shatter this bucolic scene is a naughty newt. Well, not just one, there are apparently a whole gang of them. They are eco-newts – the ones that go round causing trouble on building sites. They've not yet been served with ASBOs, but it can't be far off. If they're actually caught, that is. While I've been away they've been lying down in front of diggers, holding up the construction of a new building. I don't know who teaches them this sort of thing. I suppose with living on a university campus, the whole culture of dissent has simply become ingrained. Their spirited, yet understated, reading of *'we shall not be moved'* seems to have done the trick – I understand a newt pond is on the cards.

My employer has been extremely good to me. I've been encouraged to settle back in at my own pace. I begin by looking for my chair – obviously nicked by someone not expecting my return. I am not entitled to a 'personal' chair (this is an old university joke). Then some mouse practice. I haven't played solitaire in ages. Eventually emails and people catch up with me.

My biggest concern has been the stoma. It let me down on my first day. While talking to a colleague I'd not seen for months, it clearly became impatient – jealous even – and started gurgling, as if desperate for attention. Too much coffee I guess. I'm lucky that my office is near a disabled loo, but dealing with the bag when out is not the same as it is at home. Although I decided not to bring a spare bag, I still am a little nervous about leaks and with good reason.

Tuesday saw the first leak (since May) from my super-duper convex bag. I'd been to Oxford for a CT scan and as well as fasting beforehand I was asked to drink a litre of liquid drain-unblocker. It's very er, ... thorough – and an hour and half drive, with a seat-belt across my lap was simply too much for it and I arrived home accompanied by that old familiar warm, damp sensation.

The other major adjustment to returning to work is what to wear. I've slobbed around in post-op grunge, or a tee-shirt and shorts, all summer. I've not worn socks since May. I smarten myself up, but reserve the right to wear BIG trousers.

People tell me I look really well. This is a mixed blessing. I don't want them thinking I've been skiving for the past eight months. But I do feel well, so I don't complain.

And now my exam results...

Is it?

PET scan A*
CT scan A*

Meaning I go through to meet the liver surgeon in round two.

Or ...

I fail chemotherapy and go back six squares.

It's ... (sound of envelope tearing) ...

A*s all round. Result.

So liver tumour – prepare to meet thy doom.

I celebrate by playing a gig in a pub overlooking the Grand Union canal; I have fun – I feel alive in a way I haven't experienced before. I know it's not over yet – I still have two operations to get through – but it feels like the end is in sight. I think, as the sun sets over the water, that I am a very lucky man.

My celebration is complete when later that night, courtesy of my good friends Jenny and Steve, I become the proud owner of a motorcycle – a Harley-Davidson 1200 *Sportster*. The very one. But at a scale of 1:18 it will probably suit the newts more than me. On seconds thoughts, no – the last thing work needs is a gang of Hell's Newts terrorising the place.

I would just like to wish you all the best for this upcoming operation and I sincerely hope that you make a full recovery. Your blog really is an inspiration to others and reading your thoughts makes me realise how lucky I am to be fit and healthy. I look forward to reading your future comments and hope that pictures of you in a kilt are not uploaded any time soon ;-)

Take Care and God Bless, Craig
8th September 2006

Hi Ian, it's quite a relief to be able to talk to someone who is experiencing almost the same as me! I was diagnosed in May 2001 with colon cancer which had metastasised to my liver, only mine has decided to separate into lots of tiny tumours all over the show!! I had two lots of chemo and because the little horrors had shrunk I was able to take part in a clinical trial at Leicester which was brilliant. It seemed to do the trick so I was fortunate to be able to have a liver resection and have my remaining little friends microwaved in November 2004. I was then declared cancer free!!!!! I remained on the trial as a backup until June 2005 but unfortunately some of the little darlings must have been playing tricks as the cancer returned and the drugs decided to forsake me, so I had to quit the trial. Guess what – more chemo, what joy, three months of feeling lousy but thanking my lucky stars for wonderful friends and family to keep me cheerful. So now I visit Leicester every three months for check-ups and I'm keeping well. So good luck with your op; I'll keep my fingers and everything else crossed for you and look forward to reading your next report.

Heather
11th September 2006

Action stations

September 12th 2006

It came in under the radar like an exocet. Just after the part about *'The tumour appears to be smaller than last time we looked ...'*. I'm still taking this in when the doctor carries on *'... and the hot spot on your pelvis we noticed last time seems to have gone'.* Hot spot? Pelvis? Noticed? Seems to have gone? This is all news to me. They explain it may have been an artefact of the bowel surgery. Hmm.

I don't let this dampen my spirits one bit. I'm too pleased at the thought of no more chemo. *'Unless of course it recurs'* says the consultant ...

I have the green light for the liver op – a left hemi-ectomy – and the date is confirmed: admission on October 2nd and surgery on the 3rd. Three weeks – there's a lot to do.

First a few phone calls. The PICC line has to come out before surgery. I call the oncology centre at Northampton and they agree to do it tomorrow. I shall be so relieved to get this thing out of my arm. Annie takes a photo for posterity. I arrange to see the Bag Lady for a stoma make-over at the end of the month.

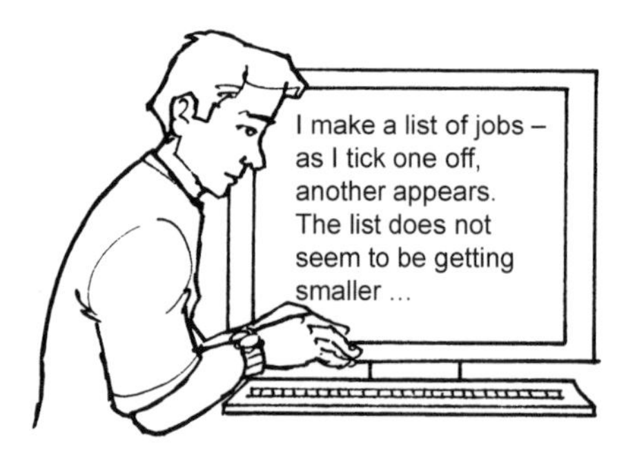

I make a list of jobs – as I tick one off, another appears. The list does not seem to be getting smaller (unlike my tumour).

My weight has increased: I'm now 14st which is the heaviest I've ever been – the result of poor diet and lack of exercise. It's all accumulating around the middle. This not only reduces my overall level of fitness, it's causing problems for my stoma. It expands just as I do, but I've not increased the size of the hole in the bag. As a result I strangle the stoma – not a pleasant experience.

I resolve to lose some weight over the next three weeks. I trim my beard and lose a few grams (well, every little helps).

I'm asked to take part in a clinical trial for a new drug. Hmm – clinical trial – wasn't there something in the news recently about clinical trials? I agree in principle, but take some documentation home to read. They're testing a drug to be administered alongside chemo drugs. The idea is that it shuts down the patient's DNA allowing the chemo drugs to be more effective. To test its efficacy they need a fresh tumour. Timing is critical – there's a window of only 12 hours between taking the drug and surgery. My only real concern is that the timing might jeopardise my operation. I'm assured that surgery has priority.

I talk it over with Annie. It won't affect my treatment in any way – I'm done with chemo. But the treatments I've had to date have all been tested, in one way or another, on other people first. We both agree that I have to do it. I call the hospital to confirm.

The sun is shining and I'm not at work today. I get the bike out. I'm not ready for my racing bike – so a gentle potter along cycle paths will be sufficient for now. Well that's the idea. I set off in completely the opposite direction to the one I had in mind. I soon reach a short, but steep hill. Instead of spinning in a low gear and taking it easy, I decide to test the legs and so I'm out of the saddle pushing a big gear. My legs are like jelly when I reach the top. But for every up, there's a down and I'm soon flying down the other side – no hands. It's a test of a good bike to ride no-handed, it means the bike is perfectly set up and balanced. I'm having fun. I soon pay for it though.

On the next hill (sitting down and spinning) I can hear panting behind and I catch a glimpse of another cyclist over my shoulder. I reach the top first then head down and into a big gear. I assume I've left him gasping – I certainly am. After a few miles I'm starting to suffer – it's 28°C and as I didn't expect to ride so far or so hard, I have no water or food. Cycling is one of the few exercises where you have to eat as you do it, if not you get the 'bonk' – glycogen deficiency. I don't bother with sports snacks when I'm riding hard, a fig roll every 20 minutes or so usually does the trick. I have three circuits that I regularly ride on my racing bike – I don't measure distance or time taken – my preferred currency is fig rolls, viz: one fig roll, two fig rolls and, the longest one, three fig rolls.

I call my friend Steve to check that he's home and swing by his house for a drink. There's a long drag up to his house – it's hardly noticeable in the car, but by the time I'm near the top I'm in the granny gear and panting. I played three gigs at the weekend, but my lungs have not had this sort of work out since last year.

The way back is even harder and I'm soaking with sweat by the time I get home. I've done around ten miles. Nothing compared with Jane Tomlinson's Ride across America, but it's a start.

There's a letter waiting for me – another instalment in the Dept of Work and Pensions saga. This is going to run longer than *Lost* or *24*. I have a very terse letter (a final reminder no less) threatening to stop my Incapacity Benefit unless I submit a medical certificate. But I'm not getting any benefit – which is why I've gone back to work. Since receiving a letter notifying me that my entitlement to IB has been turned down, I've had one letter explaining that my benefit will be taxed and two demanding medical certificates. I can't decide whether to reply or ignore it. I guess it will all depend on how my list of jobs progresses.

I email work to let them know I shall be off again, from the beginning of October. The recovery period is expected to be around eight to ten weeks. I ask them to reserve a place for me at the Christmas lunch. I'll have the turkey, but I'll forgo the liver pâté.

You have 'only' the one in your liver then? That's soon to be fried too! Good going Ian! You'll be up and around after your operation next month before you know it. You'll be cancer free too by the sounds of it – apart from maybe one or two mop up sessions of chemo?? – fingers crossed! As soon as you are able, let us all know how the operation has gone won't you? Mum and Dad are enjoying Canada! Now visiting the USA and Cowboy Country I believe and Mount Rushmore! I think Dad'll be back at the hospital November/December time for a CT scan to check on things and then more than likely it'll be another session of treatment but as long as it keeps him alive and here with us all, then that is what must be done.

Cath
12th September 2006

It's great to see regular updates appearing on your blog despite how much you have to occupy you over the coming weeks. You have such a talent for writing and I hope that the blog continues for a while after the full recovery! I really did laugh at your blog from 9th September, spirits are clearly up and I'm sure your positive outlook is helping to speed your recovery. Oh and thanks for the reply earlier this month, very amusing!

Take care, Craig
14th September 2006

Lost for words

September 25th 2006

For the first time since I started this blog I seem to be lost for words, I feel as if I have nothing much to say. Given this diary is as much for my benefit as anything else, this is a bit of a worry. I mention it to Annie and she's not surprised – *'You're well now, back to normal'.* Can it be that simple? Seems logical – no point in continually writing *'Dear diary – am feeling normal today'.*

I bought a new notebook the day I was diagnosed, to record my thoughts. For the first couple of weeks I wrote it up conscientiously every night, recording the minutiae of my day. Then the gaps started to appear. Instead of my thoughts it became a repository for appointments, or lists of things to do. It returned to its former role once in hospital, but again tailed off towards the end. At first I put this down to fatigue, boredom, etc. Anything but my aptitude as a diarist. Then I remember another attempt aged nine. That started off along the following *lines 'Got up, fed the dog, went to school'.* Another entry; *'Came home from school. Hate Mr C-. (Mr C-?). Played with Bobby (the dog). Went to bed'.* You get the picture. Not exactly a resource for generations to come, but it was a start.

My career as the new Samuel Pepys was short lived however. I felt, at age nine, that there was only so much I could say about school and my dog. And Mr C-. Although, now I think about him, there is a lot more I could say. About Mr C- that is. And school.

As for Bobby, he was a border collie named for Black Bob, canine hero of *The Dandy* and faithful companion of shepherd Andrew Glenn. My dad, cycling home from work one night, found a puppy trapped in a fence and bought it home. I can still remember the small black and white head poking out from my dad's raincoat. We asked around but no one claimed him so he became our/my dog. Unfortunately we knew nothing about vaccinations back then and he eventually died of distemper after about a year. I cried my heart out.

But what else to say? I guess it's a bit like forums (fora, sorry) for consumer products – people only write when there's a problem. No one writes to say they've been using a product for years and never experienced any of the problems others seem to have. A case of 'the squeaky wheel gets the grease?' So I guess Annie must be right. If it were not for the impending operation and this thing stuck to my stomach I would, to all intents and purposes, be back to normal. The effects of chemo seem long gone – no more Mr Yellow Tongue – although Mr Grumpy seems to have put in an appearance of late. I feel fine – not as fit as I was this time last year and a few pounds heavier (quite a few in fact), but I feel healthy. Seems absurd with a tumour on my liver.

My brain however, is not in the same place as my body. I'm feeling wobbly as I count down to surgery. I had five weeks' notice; the first week I was scared, the next two to three relaxed and happy, but this past week stressed and anxious. I know what to expect this time. In a week or so, I'm going to be vulnerable and dependant. To go into hospital, independent, in control of my life, and then to surrender seems so unreal, particularly as I'm feeling fine; like a backward step.

My stay in hospital will be different this time in one important respect; it's a 100 mile round trip – or three hours' travelling – so visiting will not be easy. I'm stocking up on books and charging up my *iPod*. This is where the proposed NHS reforms break down for me. I, like many others I guess, want a local hospital (just like we want good local schools). I can understand the rationale for wanting to create centres of excellence, but I wonder if those who plan them have spent weeks away from family and friends in an environment of fear and anxiety. The argument is broadly about improving patient care and patient choice (what choice? – when asked I bet most people would prefer local to distant care). But patient care is not solely determined by technical facilities or advanced skills – it also embraces soft options like access to, and for, loved ones.

I know it's not as simple as that – I want the best treatment and I want it on my doorstep. I want it both ways. That goes with the territory, I'm afraid. Cancer, like any other life-threatening illness, is not only an assault on the body: it attacks relationships, work, leisure, financial well-being and the mind, in fact every aspect of life. And now, having started off with nothing to say, I find I'm repeating myself, as readers of earlier entries will no doubt testify. Is that due to cancer, or age, I wonder?

Hospital beds are not kind to the muscles – I'm told that we lose 4% of our muscle mass for every 24 hours spent on a ventilator. And those recovering from liver surgery tend to go straight to intensive care as a matter of course. After my last stay in hospital I could only walk with a stick, so as a precaution I get out on the bike as much as I can. I even manage a ride on my racing bike; ten miles – piece of cake. (That's an allusion to my state of mind, rather than what I ate while riding. Although with the right sort of cake I might easily have done 20. Now that really would be something to write about.)

'Back to normal?' … sounds like yes and no. Back on your bike and playing in the band, but then this big operation ahead … maybe 'daunting' … how does that word fit what you are feeling? I cannot state exactly what you are feeling, I can only guess at it. I feel I can identify with the concept of having got over one operation plus adjuvant treatments (the famous cut, poison and burn regimes), to face a series of operations of which one was very extensive with a long recovery period. I was highly reluctant to give up the normality I had clawed back for myself. It was like walking back into the lion's den.
'To go into hospital, independent, in control of my life, and then to surrender seems so unreal, particularly as I'm feeling fine; like a backward step.'
All the best Ian, and by that I mean, all the best that it can be – 'cos I cannot deny that it sounds like it is going to be a big operation.

Take care, JJ
26th September 2006

Your operation will go well Ian, no doubt about that, what you need to try and focus on is the fact that after it, you'll be cancer free – remission is a possibility for you – ultimately you are a 'lucky' one. Mum and Dad went to Canada and USA, had to come back a week early as

Dad began to go a bit yellow – jaundiced! Having ultrasound tomorrow, they think a tumour is pushing on something and blocking his bile duct area, the nurses said it is not how big it is but where it is. He may have to go back onto chemo too which is a real bummer as he's only been off it eight or nine weeks. Another of the nurses said 'not to panic, it is quite common and a stent may have to be put in'. Bloody hell – why my Dad, why you, both fit and generally healthy men?? Life is not fair and this disease is not fair, no-one deserves it, especially my Dad, how long will he go on for? Well, stage 4 – no stats really except stage 3 only 15% make it to two years – help – I feel a breakdown coming on. I cannot imagine how you and your loved ones are coping because I know that I am not very well, I keep getting this awful dread feeling in the pit of my stomach – what if Dad's not here soon, etc. You will be another success story and statistic of beating this disease and for that you need to be eternally grateful, you are an inspiration to others, try not to worry too much about the op, big one, yes I know, but you are back on the road to recovery now and that bodes well for your future. I look forward to more updates from you as always. xxx.

Cath
27th September 2006

Hi Ian, Just wanted to say good luck and offer some reassurance. I had my own liver resection on 1st August. Like you I was very anxious and was prepared for a lengthy recovery. Whilst it wasn't exactly a walk in the park, it was not as bad as I feared. Eight weeks on I am mobile, driving and feeling generally OK. In fact, I have recovered more quickly from this than I did from my original bowel op in January. I really hope all goes well for you and this message helps a little with the nerves.

Suemac
27th September 2006

The dark side of the Moon

September 29th 2006

One of the most dramatic aspects of the Apollo Moon programme was the lunar orbit. For about two hours those back on Earth held their collective breath as the lunar module disappeared behind the Moon – severing all contact. Cheers and tears greeted the astronauts when they finally emerged from this temporary exile. Was the anxiety misplaced? The lunar module was just as vulnerable during its nearside orbits as it was during those on the far side. We just didn't know what was happening once we had lost contact. Imagination takes over. Is the danger any less because we can see it? Probably not at that distance.

I too will be out of touch for a while. My own journey to the dark side carries an element of risk. But there's a greater risk if I don't go. A rock and a hard place? That's probably over simplifying things – a rock and a hard place implies an element of choice. Which I don't have. I'm not in the business of weighing up risks – I shall not read the consent form, merely sign it. And I don't gamble (much) having never done the football pools, bet on a horse or even bought a lottery ticket. Although as a child in Scotland, I did occasionally act as a bookie's runner for my grandmother, taking wee notes down to the man in the billiards hall. I had no idea what I was doing and the Polis wadnae suspect a polite and shy English schoolboy.

So am I gambling now? I'm convinced the cancer will spread if left untreated. So the operation looks, on the face of it, a no-brainer. I just hope that's not how I end up.

It's all about trust. I trust the medical team to do their jobs. That's not to say I'm expecting perfection. Things go wrong as I know only too well. Trust means defining roles and responsibilities. I had occasion to talk to a factory manager about his management philosophy. He put it very succinctly: *'If you give people responsibility, you've got to accept their decision-making'*. I adopted this as my creed both at work and as a parent. It's a tough one to follow, particularly when dealing with children, or if you don't like delegating, but I believe in it.

I've given the medical team responsibility for removing my tumour. If they say surgery is the best way of dealing with my particular situation, then so be it. This does not mean that I sit back and let others get on with it, far from it – I've done all I can to get fit and keep healthy, in order to give them the best chance of success. And I read up about treatments so that I can have a meaningful conversation with them. It's a partnership – they do their bit and I do mine.

New treatments and breakthroughs are emerging all the time. I've just been reading an article in the Daily Mail[ii] about a team at the

Leicester Royal Infirmary who are using microwaves to treat tumours on the liver. Sounds promising, but a bit messy for the average kitchen, and there's no mention of what setting to use or how long to leave it in for.

There is still a lot to do as countdown approaches. Manage to fit in a haircut – to my surprise, my hair, having thinned a little during chemo, is now growing back very thickly. Even so, I can't really endorse chemo as a solution for the folically challenged.

Also manage to fit in a visit to the Bag Lady for a 'Stoma Wax and Polish'. My stoma has changed size yet again. This time it's smaller than the cut-out on the bag, causing irritation to the skin. As usual she sorts it out and my stoma sparkles and gleams like new.

In the post today a further episode in the Department of Work & Pensions saga. This time (the sixth missive since this sorry affair began) they inform me that I meet 'the threshold of incapacity'. Which is quite timely as I'm about to stop work for the next three months or so. But they still won't pay, as I don't meet the financial criteria – having an occupational pension disqualifies me. However, it is a comfort to know that my cancer treatment is considered serious enough to keep me from working. I try telephoning to ask why they keep writing to me, but it's busy as usual. Can I be bothered to write? Nah. Too much else to do.

Having taken what I consider to be a completely logical and rational approach to my cancer treatment, I then realise I am not consistent. I'm glad not to be having surgery this month – I don't like Septembers, never have. This is not superstition but something that goes back to my school days. September lies; it promises a new beginning (eg. start of a new school year) – but all around things are starting to whither and die. The sun was shining when I went back to work. On my days off, especially those that were warm, I went out on my bike. But all around, the signs and smells of autumn – made worse this year by the sight of dying horse chestnut trees, perhaps as big a threat as dutch elm disease was 30 years ago.

October is a much more straightforward month – a sort of 'what you see is what you get' type of month. It can still be warm, but there's no denying that the days are getting shorter. I'm not unhappy to be going into orbit during October.

I'm reassured, and touched – humbled even – by the messages of support and comments on my blog. So, I raise a last glass of red wine to send my liver on its way, and it's off to the launch pad.

À bientôt. TTFN. Later.

Oh – here goes – 'blast off' approaching Ian, all the very best for a successful operation and speedy recovery so we can all get back to reading your fantastic thoughts/feelings and supporting each other. May God go with you and your family at this time.

Cath

29th September 2006

[11] *My tumour was microwaved away*. Daily Mail (online) September 26th 2006 (http://www.dailymail.co.uk/pages/live/articles/health/healthmain.html?in_article_id=406955&in_page_id=1774)

Déjà-vu

October 2nd – 9th 2006

I've been here before. Last time it was fatigue, this time it's pain. I have a technique – roll on to my side, let my legs drop off the side of the bed and then push up with my arms. A combination of gravity and muscle swings me upright and I'm sitting on the edge of the bed. Only now I'm stuck. I can't get off the bed. Annie tries to take my arm, but it's no good – the pain is excruciating. I manage a clumsy reverse and sink back onto the bed, gasping for breath.

It's Friday afternoon – three days after surgery. I wanted to show off my progress to Annie: yesterday afternoon, I had not only got out of bed but managed a walk as well.

On the Friday morning ward round one of the doctors said I could go home on Saturday. The drain and catheter were taken out and the epidural removed. It's the removal of the epidural that brings me up short – no pain relief. The consultant comes to see me in the evening. He's unhappy at the idea of me going home on Saturday – *'That's a big wound'* – he wants me to wait until Monday. I'm happy with this, I need to get an alternative to the epidural sorted out. But progress is still much quicker than I expected, especially given how slowly the week started.

Monday October 2nd

I ring at noon to find out if there's a bed free. No luck yet – they'll ring back. As the afternoon wears on I feel deflated. I've psyched myself up to going and have been feeling positive, but the waiting eats into my mood. I try again at 4.00pm. Still no joy. I eventually get a call at 4.50pm: there's a bed free in a short stay ward. I can have that until my operation.

We arrive about 6.30pm and meet up with the doctor conducting the clinical trial. I'm second on the list for surgery, which means I should go down to theatre around mid-morning. I'm to have the drugs at midnight. I sign a consent form and then settle down to wait. Annie goes about 8.00; suddenly it's all very quiet.

Around 9.30 I'm aware of a young girl at the side of my bed. She wants to know why I'm having liver surgery. I'm a bit confused as to who she is. She has a stethoscope and at first I assume it's 'take your daughter to work' day. I can't believe she's a doctor – she looks so young. But after an expert examination, it's clear I've misjudged her. I'm getting old.

Tuesday October 3rd

Alarms go off around 4.00am and there's pandemonium. A cardiac arrest somewhere on the ward. I count about 20 people running past my bed. Eventually it all calms down. I'm calm too – I'm not nervous any more about the operation.

An anaesthetist comes by around 8.00 to explain about 'pain management'. He says I'll be left with what they call the 'Mercedes Scar' – three lines radiating out from my middle like the logo of a German motorcar.

Mid-morning and there's a trio of young ladies standing at the foot of the bed. I find myself staring and they giggle. I expect them to burst into '*Three little maids from school are we*', instead they tell me they are part of the 'surgical team'. It's hard to explain just how young these doctors seem to me. It's like my own children were preparing to hack in to me. If this were a TV show I'd be in an episode of *Scrubs*, rather than *Casualty* or *Holby City*.

I'm given a pair of surgical stockings to put on. They're full length. I start to roll them up my leg (as I've seen done in many a film) and get a very funny look from a couple of visitors passing my bed. It's noon and it's all gone quiet again. The operation is delayed. The waiting is hard – it's as if I reach a peak of mental preparation, which then dissipates and I have to start again. They finally come for me at 2.00pm.

The anaesthetist turns out to be a bike rider – he's ridden the Alps this summer. As the epidural goes in, he talks about climbing the *Alpe d'Huez*, one of the most dramatic stages of the *Tour de France*...

... and the next thing I know, I'm being woken by a nurse. It's around 9.00pm and it's all over. I'm in the recovery room – not Intensive Care. I've lost over four pints of blood and about 40% of my liver but I'm doing OK. No leaking from the bile duct. Blood loss on this sort of scale is not uncommon for those who've had chemo. I had visions of it spurting out and people sticking their fingers in the holes – I guess that's just plain silly though. Four pints is about half the average adult volume – no wonder I look pale from the waist up. The tumour was about 50mm long. At around 10.00 they take me up to the ward and to a waiting Annie. This is such a change from last time.

Wednesday October 4th

The numbers are good – blood pressure, heart rate and respiration. I've been on oxygen overnight, but I take it off. I have a drain on my left side, but the level seems to have stabilised. My clean respiration is cause for much comment, it's very common for fluid to build in the lungs when you're in bed for any length of time. I had a sing-song with a bunch of musician friends on Saturday night and I'm convinced that that, along with all the bike riding, have given my lungs a thorough spring clean.

I manage to sit in the chair by my bed for about half an hour. My shoulders are painful – this is referred pain from the diaphragm which came in for some man-handling during the operation. Referred pain is not amenable to the epidural so I'm given paracetamol. Late evening my temperature spikes and a call is put through to the doctor on call. I have a mild panic – this is just what happened last time.

The ward comprises a central corridor with bays off, each containing four beds. Next to me is Mr Very Offensive who swears and curses, to himself and at the nurses, continually, and opposite are two elderly ladies. One of the ladies has the most incredible night-time 'turns' – she talks in her sleep: it starts coherently enough but then turns into what I can only describe as 'speaking in tongues'. I listen intently trying to make out any recognisable words or phrases, but it all passes me by. I've never heard anything like it. It drives everybody – patients and staff – mad. She's given injections at night to help her sleep but all this does is ensure that she sleeps through the daytime as well. She has severe respiratory problems and her oxygen mask and nebuliser serve to amplify the sound to something approaching Darth Vader. This night is, apparently, a particularly bad one. At around 2.00am Mr Very Offensive starts shouting at her – I can understand his frustration but he becomes very offensive. This, of course, has no effect: the poor woman is fast asleep, so he turns his television on at full volume and now everyone's awake. After a slanging match between him and the night staff, his bed is moved to the end of the corridor. I must ask Annie to bring in earplugs.

Thursday October 5th

The drain is taken out and the dressings are changed. The wound is stapled. My Mercedes scar looks more like how a child would draw a railway line (albeit a railway line that runs along the San Andreas fault). The wound is looking so good that the dressings are left off and I have a small patch over the drain hole. I'm allowed lunch from the 'soft/moist' menu – soup (no roll), jelly and ice-cream.

Mid afternoon the physio comes to take me for a walk. To his surprise and mine, I manage a walk to the end of the ward and back. *This is one small step for a man ...* The physio feels confident that he can sign me off there and then – no need for any more visits from him.

Having made good his escape, the bed previously occupied by Mr Very Offensive is now home to a young woman. She snores all night. Forget hospital food, forget super bugs – it's the noise that really gets to you.

Friday October 6th

The epidural has been a great success. A background level of pain-killer is administered by drip and then I top it up myself via a hand control, as and when needed. It's stayed in for the duration – last time it leaked after a couple of days and I went on to morphine. The epidural is taken out at lunchtime – and once it's taken out it cannot be put back in. I have a visit from the pain management team – they're concerned that I may be discharged within 24 hours of an epidural coming out. This is not a good idea apparently. I top myself up just before it's disconnected but by the time Annie arrives (around 5.00) the effects are wearing off and the alternative will not be administered for a couple of hours yet. Which is why I get stuck in bed. *Déjà-vu* indeed.

Annie can't find any earplugs so brings a pair of ear defenders (industrial size) and I get my first complete night's sleep since I've been here. The nurses laugh, but I don't care. These are top of my list of 'things to bring for your stay in hospital'.

Saturday/Sunday October 7/8th

The weekend passes slowly. I now have a mix of pills for pain relief – some make me sick, some don't. I ask not to be put on morphine and am given *Tramadol* instead. Over the course of the day my reaction fluctuates; I also lose my appetite.

Three members of the band visit on Saturday afternoon and they tell me how well I look. I tell them I now have a Mercedes – (can't resist it) – and lift up my gown to prove it.

I have to change the stoma bag. This turns out to be tricky as it's awkward trying to do this in a hospital bed and the middle part of my body is completely numb. There is no feeling from my lower abdomen to my chest. So I can't feel the stoma when I try to clean it. It's bizarre.

I'm woken early on Sunday morning (six-ish) for blood pressure and temperature readings and am aware that I feel no pain or nausea whatsoever. But by the time breakfast arrives I can't eat it. I'm taken off the 'soft/moist' menu and lunch is roast pork. I know there are so many jokes about hospital food and to be fair, some of it is quite good, but what arrives on my plate looks just like one of those rubber heels that my dad used for repairing our shoes. I now know where the expression 'tough as old boots' comes from. I cannot cut it with a knife – but I'm hungry so I persist and manage half of it. At least my jaws get a good work out.

Sunday afternoon and I'm up and walking when Annie arrives. By Sunday evening I can walk to the loo unaided. I'm surprised just how quickly I am recovering from this operation. It's only really the adverse affect of the pain-killers that slows me down.

Monday October 9th

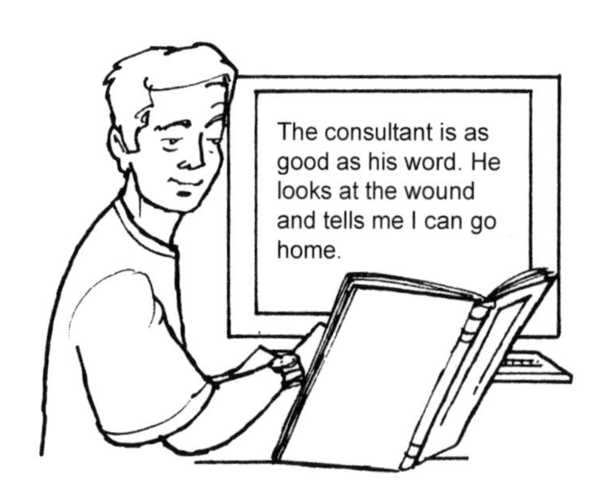

The consultant is as good as his word. He looks at the wound and tells me I can go home. Annie's not free to collect me until around 5.00pm so I settle back on the bed with a new book. Not for long though – they want the bed and I'm moved to the Discharge Lounge. I try to imagine what this is like – for some reason my mind jumps to airport departure lounges and I wonder 'economy' or 'business class'? In the event it looks like an Age Concern furniture store. A jumble of sensible high-backed armchairs, and the clientele look as if their age may be of some concern. I arrive, with others, by wheelchair. Because of the high furniture density, there is much to-ing and fro-ing and three point turns before the 'drivers' eject their charges into one of the waiting chairs. In the general mêlée I make a dash for the only bed in the room – well I'm going to be here for about six hours so I may as well be comfortable.

I'm always amazed by the elderly. Within minutes of arrival two complete strangers have struck up a conversation and know each other's age, medical history, financial and familial status. Although largely humourous, these encounters can be poignant; a widow asks a widower when his wife died. He replies; *'I don't know – I lost my memory 11 years ago'*. It reminds me of very young children who are also able to speak with such frankness and innocence.

I'm the last to leave. I have my pills (19 a day for the next two weeks) and an overwhelming sense of gratitude. By a combination of skill and luck – skill on the part of the medical staff at the John Radcliffe Hospital, Oxford and luck in the sense that the tumour was on the left side of my liver rather than the right, I have come through this operation quickly and without complication. I'm not aware of any side effects from the clinical trial. My body looks a mess – Annie says my bikini-wearing days are over, but I feel great and can't wait to get home.

I am so pleased to hear that you are doing better than last time.
Déjà-vu … yes, whenever I read your blogs that's what I think of … techniques and strategies for coping after an operation … things I just wish someone had told me beforehand. It sounds like you are coping even tho' it has been difficult, and you certainly didn't have your sense of humour removed at the same time. I am desperately trying to remember what a Mercedes badge looks like and shall have to keep my eyes open for one.
My experience of cancer has led me to believe that support doesn't always come from where you might expect. I think this is especially so when you consider the on-going nature, (further ops, treatment, fears of reoccurrence, slow return to NormalWorld, etc.) – leading to feelings of isolation and separateness for myself. Hence, it is important to me to be supportive towards others in similar situations. I am just so glad to hear you're recovering so well.

All the best JJ
16th October 2006

Wishful thinking

October 24th 2006

Strange times. The other day Annie said, *'You don't have cancer any more'.* In a way she's right, but if only it were that simple. The cancer engine was removed in January and the (only apparent) secondary of that engine was removed a couple of weeks ago. But if the removal of a tumour was the end of the story, none of us would have to go through regular testing and checkups.

The wound is healing. The staples were taken out last week – not at all painful except for those located right at the far ends of my Mercedes scar. The central area was still somewhat numb (a bit like having an injection at the dentist) and so although I was aware of the nurse pulling at the staples, any sensation felt far, far away. But at the periphery, sense is returning and I have to say, it hurt, just a little. So the railway tracks are no more; a red river valley now runs down my chest and bifurcates south-east and south-west, just below my ribs.

Annie says it looks worse now than it did when I came out of surgery. The dead centre of the wound, the point where the three scars meet is a case in point. The upper left-hand section has healed at a lower level than the other two sections – a slight landslip – only a few mm deep but noticeable all the same. Fresh from her decorating successes, she keeps offering to get the electric sander out to erode the difference. I think she's wrong; it needs *Polyfilla* to build up the lower section rather than a sander to remove healthy tissue. But I'm inclined to leave things just as they are. Bill Clinton said, after all his heart surgery, that his body was a complete mess, but that he was past caring (or words to that effect), and I feel the same. Anyway – given that it's sitting over the part of my body where the liver has been removed, I might experience some tectonic uplift as the liver grows back.

The regeneration of the liver is a weird thing. I was told that it would take around three months for my lost 40% to be replaced. Just in time for Christmas. I decide to forgo alcohol during this period to give the liver a sporting chance. But how will I know when it's regrown? How will it know when to stop? I imagined they might have left a window or a gauge so I could chart its progress.

I notice that the zits have gone from my face and my body. I have always put them down to poor diet, but clearly that cannot be the case. Was it the chemo that gave rise to these eruptions? Or the tumour on the liver? Hard to tell. It's almost impossible to remember the day some particular symptom first appeared – I became aware once chemo had started, but not before.

There is a certain amount of adjustment required post-surgery – probably more this time than last. It's this sense of 'it's all over – yet it's not all over'. Unfinished business.

Most mornings I wake up sore and have to deal with that first. But as the soreness wears off and I tune in to my surroundings, a feeling of relief and contentment sweeps over me. I am glad and lucky to be here. Others are not so.

A friend of a friend of Annie's was diagnosed with cancer in July. He passed away last weekend. And a colleague from work had a stroke from which she did not recover. Whether death is a few hours or a few months away from the first signs that something is not quite right, it is still something of a shock. We are never prepared. Although we grow up with a sneaking feeling that our parents will one day die, we are never equipped to deal with the death of a child or a friend or colleague, especially when they happen to be around the same age as ourselves. Perhaps it's something to do with the fact that death is relatively uncommon in our (Western) culture. In all my years on this planet, I've seen just three dead bodies. Television or film, however graphic, does not count. Perhaps it makes it worse – we know it's make believe.

I think this is why being told we have cancer is so shocking. It's not what we have come to expect, it only happens to other people. Perhaps a small amount of self-denial is useful – it keeps us optimistic, hoping for the best. Too much, however, and it's not just us that suffers, but those around us as well. And, as with death, we go through a period of bereavement – mourning for the loss of our old life. Things will never be the same again. And it's not just those with the disease who feel this – our loved ones, carers, supporters go through this too.

I knew so little about cancer before my diagnosis. Apart from one or two lucky souls who made the news, I saw it as a death sentence. I know better now. But I'm moving into uncharted territory. I'm off the map and into the region marked *Here There Be Dragons.* It's now down to regular monitoring, will power and luck ('but the greatest of these is luck').

So although the tumours have been removed I cannot allow myself to believe it's all over yet, although I have started looking at the odd holiday brochure with an eye to next year. In just the same way as the chemo drugs fought my cancer cells, I have this other, cerebral, battle going on. Optimists versus pessimists. Expect the best, but prepare for the worst. This encounter plays out in my head. Most days it's very one-sided. But perhaps all that I've been through so far are merely skirmishes. Maybe the big battle is yet to come. Or maybe the cancer cells will simply throw down their weapons and run away. Wishful thinking?

I suppose like you said Ian, you are now 'cancer free', some people never have that, you are a 'lucky' one to have had only one secondary and that it was in an area of liver that could be removed. I wish you and Annie all the best for a long life together – I only wish my Dad's prognosis had been as good as yours. May you start booking holidays soon and get back to living a full life!

Cath
25th October 2006

Ian I send you very big warm wishes for the future and huge, but gentle, virtual hugs. I found out about your cancer and blog through a mutual friend. I totally identify with what you've mentioned here regarding life after surgery and chemo and I have to say I found it quite scary for a long time. Having had a reprieve and a second crack at life everything was totally uncertain and I was uncomfortable about making plans or even talking about the future but hey I'm still here 12 years later and living on a Greek Island having given up everything in the UK to realise 'my dream' pre-cancer! So for me something massively fantastic came out of it. Book that holiday!!!

Take care, Gail
26th October 2006

Aches and pains. And cranes

November 1st 2006

I seem to be spending a lot of time on my back right now. I'm not yet able to sleep on my side. Sitting hunched over a computer or a guitar, for that matter, is only something I can do for a few minutes at the most. There is a sweet spot where nothing hurts which can only be found when I'm horizontal. As a consequence I am becoming something of an expert on ceilings. I'm also becoming an expert on TV shopping channels (although I don't really understand *price drop TV* – how do they make their money?).

It's been four weeks (!) since the operation and I've slid back a little in my recovery. The medication for dealing with the after-effects of surgery has made me ill; I have *Tramadol* (for pain relief) which messes up my guts, *Diclophenac* (an anti-inflammatory) which messes up my guts and *Omeprazole* (to counter the effects of the *Diclophenac*) which messes up ...

Despite the discomfort, I find the stoma fascinating. Something I've never noticed before is that stuff does not come out in the order it went in. I had assumed that the progress of food through the gut would be an orderly business – my colon is after all British and should know a thing or two about queuing – but no, it all appears to be a bit of a mad dash and Devil take the hindmost. If this appears a bit indelicate, I beg indulgence – at the moment I can only watch the ceiling, watch television or watch my bag. And it's a toss up between TV and the bag as to which has the most c**p.

I saw the consultant last week and he has taken me off everything. So now I'm a bit sore. It's a job to stand upright. I can't sing either – just can't get enough air into the lungs. Even going upstairs leaves me breathless. I feel like I did six months ago. I know it won't last long; as my bike-riding hero Lance A. is fond of saying *'pain is temporary'*. The wound is healing fine although it looks a mess – the Mercedes scar looks as if the Beastie Boys[12] have had a go at it.

It continues to surprise me just how much drugs affect our minds and bodies – probably a naïve thought to those who've been through all this. The numbness in my torso is just about gone (which is why it now hurts) but I have the strangest sensation in my feet. On the night in hospital when my temperature spiked, my right foot became numb and extremely cold. A nurse had to massage it to get any feeling back into it. Since then I have a dull numbness in the three largest toes on each foot which is almost like pins and needles, but not quite. The consultant wondered about chemo as a suspect, but as that ended three months ago, I can't quite see it myself. Given the referred pain in the shoulders from messing with the diaphragm, I can't help wondering what a reflexologist or acupuncturist would make of all this.

He also went on to explain (well, he didn't completely: *'I won't tell you exactly what we did'),* but the gist of it seemed to involve a lot of pulling and bending and clamping parts of the body which normally enjoy a relatively quiet life. He reassured me that it was quite normal to experience rapid recovery and then set backs, and it would probably take three months before I'm back to normal; *'It was a big operation'.* Unlike the liver resection shown on last night's episode of *Holby City*. Not a Mercedes scar in sight. I find this up and down bit hard to explain to other people. Just a week after leaving hospital I was sitting in a pub listening to a couple of friends making music. Everyone says I look well, they can't believe I've just had liver surgery, etc., etc.

The next stage is a check-up in three months, a scan in six months and then, assuming nothing has come back, checkups once a year for the next five years. I was somewhat surprised when the consultant mentioned that Oxford would keep an eye on me over this period – I had assumed as the primary cancer was treated at Milton Keynes, that's where any follow-ups would be. But the prospect of further trips to Oxford turns out to be, in a rather surprising way, right up Annie's street.

The Churchill Hospital in Oxford, where I go for scans and consultations, is a bit of a mess right now. A massive building programme is underway. Of particular interest to me is the planned opening next year of a *Maggie's Centre*[13] – a place where cancer patients, survivors, loved ones can go for help and advice and even just a bit of peace and quiet.

The site is visible from quite a distance, thanks to the large flock of cranes dominating the skyline. These cranes (engineering rather than avian) hold a fascination for Annie, which I am quite unable to fathom. Her excitement begins as soon as they come in to sight and increases as we make our way into the hospital. We stop at the 'Friends of Churchill' teashop and she makes a mad dash to get a window seat to continue this love affair.

The teashop is on the first floor and laid out before her is a blank canvas of trenches, mounds, piles of bricks and other assorted building material with four tower cranes (they look like the uppercase letter T) busily raising, lowering and swinging to-and-fro to some unheard and unseen choreographer. In the foreground is what she calls a 'Noddy crane' which, thanks to *Wikipedia*, we later identify as a 'tower crane with pivoted main boom' (it looks like an uppercase Y). A moment's reflection and I begin to panic. We are turning into crane-spotters. It'll be packed lunches, a Thermos and a copy of *I-SPY Building Sites* next.

These cranes fascinate Annie; *'How do they get the arm on top of the tower?'; 'How do they get the counterweight up there?'; 'How does the man know where to move it to?'*

The teashop is crowded and I fight my way to this ringside seat. After a while I start to sulk and grumble at the prospect of fighting my way out – I can't bear to be in a crowd while I have this bag attached to me; I have a fear (irrational, I know) that someone will bump into me and burst it. It's getting late for my appointment and I make to move. Annie eats her biscuit in slow-motion; *'Can I just see this last one move?'* It's like being with a six-year-old.

It all begins to make sense; the episode with the sledge-hammer and the chimney breast in the summer, a prior history of knocking down walls and a fascination for heights (abseiling, leaping out of aeroplanes, etc.). Perhaps she should have been a civil engineer rather than a maths teacher. I resolve to buy her a *Meccano* set for

Christmas – as long as it comes in pink. And this is not some cheap sexist slur on my part; all her friends will testify that she will only go outward bounding and bonding if there's somewhere to plug in her hair straighteners. In spite of all the rough stuff, she's a real girlie at heart.

Our next trip to the Churchill is scheduled for January – which gives me plenty of time to find the Thermos.

I am slowly reading backwards from when I first saw your blog and so come rather lately to comment on this entry ('The fact of the matter', June 30th). It sounded like a hard decision for you to part with your dog and acknowledge needing to make some changes in your life, whilst considering both your needs and also those of Annie, who might have had to take care of the dog as well as you. We used to have cats, a number of years ago, and I would have liked them there for company and cuddles when I was recuperating. I was fortunate enough to have an intermittent feline garden visitor who seemed to have limitless cuddles to share. I felt quite mutilated after my surgery and welcomed the feeling of acceptance by a gentle three-legged cat. Ah, the D-word. Cancer brought all sorts of new words that one day I sat mulling it over. I now knew what an oncologist was ... should I ever get to a social occasion and have the opportunity to show off my enlarging vocabulary. I even sat composing a Cancer Alphabet as in A is for Axilla, B is for Breast, C is for Cancer and D is for... I decided to stop at that point. Have your ever heard of the notion of there being an elephant in the room? (Maybe E can be for Elephant). Cancer can be like there being an elephant in the room and NOBODY mentioning it! I think death can be like that too. Statistically even if I can intellectualise my odds, one of the very first thoughts in my head when told of my cancer was 'Am I going to die' and 'How soon? Have I got 'til my birthday or perhaps Xmas?' I didn't ask but I thought it, and I suspect many others do too. I wonder whether people think that if you mention the word it makes it happen? If so, does that mean I must have been yattering my head off about cancer for ages to have got it to happen to me? I suspect a control issue operates like the 'be positive' one. If I don't think about it then it won't happen – a huge denial defence system operating. What the sad outcome can be is that the cancer patient feels it is hard to raise the subject of their fears for acknowledgement or discussion and carry it within, whilst also feeling they have to appear utterly positive at all times – 'cos that's what will keep the cancer away??? I am fortunate to have one or two people who will talk death with me, mine as well as theirs as well as in general. My wish is to have a commemorative bench. I hate those that say stuff about 'George, died after a long battle'. What about how they LIVED! What about who they were, or how they were loved. My friend knows I want a bench to say something like 'JJ was a good snogger and often did it here'.

JJ
10th November 2006

[12] A popular beat combo with a penchant for using automobile logos as jewellery.
[13] http://www.maggiescentres.org.uk

Moving on

November 16th 2006

I've come to a realisation that I (and I guess others with this disease) move in a different plane from those without it. I seem to inhabit the vertical plane, the rest of the world, the horizontal. Almost every day for the past year I've had to confront my own mortality, to stand on the edge peering over, and then to pull back. No wonder I'm up and down.

But life goes on and it's proving much harder to join in again than I thought it would. While I've been on sabbatical, the point of departure – the place where I temporarily left the world – is no longer there. It's moved on down the road. And I guess it's unreasonable to expect it to wait for me. It's a bit like being Einstein's time traveller. Everyone has aged in my absence.

I'm not talking about personal relationships, rather situations where we have responsibilities and roles to play – particularly if those roles and responsibilities have been shared out among others in our absence. It's no one's fault – it's simply yet another consequence of this disease. I sometimes think I may be guilty of making a special case for cancer – surely all life-threatening diseases must cause the same problems? Well, cancer is the only one I know about – but there is, to my mind, something different about this disease. It's so easy, apart from the immediate effects of treatment, to appear 'normal' to the outside world. Indeed, trying to get back to normality is an important part of the armoury for defeating this thing. When people say; *'you're looking great'* they are, quite reasonably, responding to the outward signs – they have no idea what is going on inside. I've seen and felt things that I would not wish on anyone.

Work will be a big challenge when I return after Christmas. Although I went back for a few weeks in September before liver surgery, that was mainly to clear up my desk and use up some annual leave. Not a time for anything productive. I can access my work email from home and I dip in from time to time to see what's going on. But so much has changed in my absence I could be eaves-dropping on a completely different organisation. I've missed being part of a team. I wonder how sports people feel when they miss a season through injury. It's heartening to see Kylie Minogue back on stage. Although she's not so much part of a team – she *is* the team.

Sometimes work seems trivial compared with cancer. Of course it puts a roof over my head and food on the table – it's more to do with the day-to-day challenges. In the grand scheme of things, decisions I make or tasks I perform are not in the same league as getting up each morning and overcoming demons. Not that I have to do that every day, but they've been around more than usual of late.

To my surprise I discover I feel the same about rejoining the band. Although I've played the occasional gig this year I've felt more like a guest than an original member. The show must go on and all that. I've missed rehearsals and again being part of a team.

I've always been a team player – shame we can't treat cancer in this way – *'I'll take the bowel, you have the liver and Fred can deal with the bag'.* No matter how good your supporters are cancer is still an individual event.

It's been seven weeks now since the operation and the pain is almost gone, but I'm still very sore – it's like have a belt done up too tight. My feet are still 'numb' and I begin to wonder if this all shouldn't have gone by now (someone's just emailed to say that they had a similar experience after an epidural). And I wonder about the clinical trial – re-reading the notes I should have been monitored for four weeks after surgery, but I've not heard a thing.

It's so easy to become a hypochondriac – every little thing takes on epic proportions. A pain in the neck means that my cancer has now spread to the lymph nodes. Perhaps this is just a normal part of the recovery process. I know of a few people who've had counselling after treatment for cancer and I'm beginning to understand why. Post-treatment stress disorder?

And if all this wasn't bad enough, I've just read that the risk of dying in hospital as a result of medical error is 1 in 300 – the risk of dying in an air crash, by way of comparison, is 1 in 10,000,000[14]. So if my cancer comes back I'm going to have my next surgery at 30,000 feet.

The more I think about it, the more I realise that perhaps I should have my head examined. The most bizarre thing happened on Sunday morning. I woke up with a poem in my head — fully formed, words and rhyme. OK — I won't elevate it to the status of High Art — more a set of verses. And it's certainly not profound — just nonsense. But where did it come from? I lay awake for ages mulling this over. I cannot think of anything that would have stimulated this. No book or television programme comes to mind. Perhaps there really is a Muse. I nudge Annie and although bleary-eyed, she pays attention; *'You should write that down'*. As I sit at the computer I change a couple of words. And that's it.

I hope it's original and not something I've heard in the distant past, because although dredging up something from the far recesses of our minds is quite a feat in itself, for something completely original to pop into our heads from out of nowhere, uninvited, is utterly amazing. Over the next few days, more 'poems' arrive — all fashioned within minutes. What is going on? Are the drugs still lurking around? Or is it a kind of defence mechanism — a diversion? — the brain's equivalent of putting its hands over its ears and going *'la, la, I can't hear you'*, when faced with the enormity of bringing the body back from the edge.

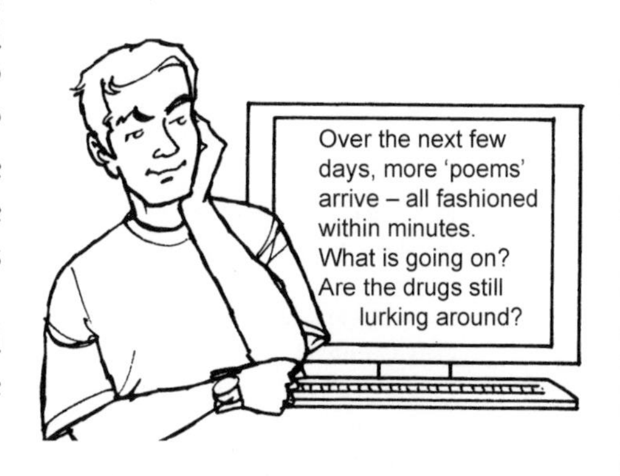

It seems to me there are three outcomes to this disease: (i) it goes into remission (maybe even cured?) (ii) it reappears in its original location or (iii) it appears in a new site. This is the burden that the cancer survivor carries — no matter how normal they appear to be. And moving on while carrying this burden is the biggest challenge. No wonder the brain wants a day off from the serious stuff.

Benny

Benny was a boxer
And a rubbish one at that
In 30 fights he'd won just once
The rest he'd been knocked flat

He'd shuffle and he'd wobble
And dance like he was pissed
Till his chin fulfilled its destiny
With his opponent's fist

He thought he'd make the big time
And be a star on telly
But you can't be a winner
With legs that work like jelly

So now he opens village fêtes
Garden Centres and the like
And instead of swanky limousines
He goes home on his bike

OK Doctor Freud, I'm ready.

Just re-reading, and your comment about cancer being an individual event struck home. Cancer has given me a set of experiences which many of my friends and family are aware of to varying (usually much lesser) extents, leading to a feeling of isolation or disconnectedness due to such different perspectives that it affords. When people said I looked well I felt so betrayed by my body's outward signs as inside was so different. Also, they were generally only seeing me when I felt well enough, so they didn't see me at my worst.
Your comment about hypochondria and ailments taking epic proportions puts me in mind of the Peter Harvey article ('After treatment finishes – then what?' www.ctrust.org.uk/article3.htm) as he speaks of having to re-learn about the body and trying to regain trust in it. Was it John Diamond who said he never had headaches, only brain tumours? The symptoms, niggles, aches that we would have ignored in the past can appear as sinister portents. Swollen lymph nodes in the neck are not due to colds or toothache, aching hip/abdominal pain are bone cancer or ovarian cancer at least.
I wonder if you have ever read Terry Pratchett books? 'Guards! Guards!' finds the City watchmen planning to kill a dragon by getting their best archer to fire his lucky arrow at the dragon's 'vulnerables', just like all the heroes do. Then they suddenly realise they don't know where its 'vulnerables' are … and also, isn't it when things are really impossible that they always happen? So they spend time trying to lengthen the odds … standing on one leg, aiming over the

shoulder, etc., etc. to try to get the odds to one in a million 'cos everyone knows that when it's one in a million then it happens nine out of ten times!! (Hope you understand stats enough to get that one.) So, perhaps we all need to ask for our ops doing at 300,000 feet by a blindfolded surgeon ... suggestions welcomed ...

JJ
17th November 2006

[14] *When surgery goes wrong*; The Independent, November 14th 2006.

It's not over till the Bag Lady rings

November 25th 2006

'You look remarkable'. There's an emphasis on 'remarkable'. This from my GP. I see him because my feet are still numb and it may be due to the epidural and it's now starting to get a little uncomfortable when I walk. I want some advice and reassurance, but both are in short supply. He confirms the epidural as the most likely candidate – but instead of a likely end date he says that it may never go. There's not a lot he can do except to suggest anti-depressants. *'But I'm not depressed'.* He assures me they're used as a mild pain-killer. Groan. Sort out the symptoms, not the cause. He's more helpful than he sounds – he was the one who sent me off pronto to see a consultant last year; but for his quick diagnosis my situation might be a lot worse.

I'm not depressed (am I?), – but I am fed up. This can be a very lonely disease. Despite the best efforts of friends and family, we still spend endless hours on our own, whether receiving, or recovering from, treatment. At times like these I spend a lot of time living inside my head. Apart from the medics, no one knows more about my cancer than me. Sometimes I go to dark places or have dark thoughts – I see the mind as an attic – I simply like to go in and have a good poke around. I find it easier to cope if I know all the possibilities, all the potential outcomes – but I didn't see this feet thing coming.

I'm also bored. So bored that I eventually succumb to the torture that is the TV shopping channels – *'OK, OK I'll buy the lateral thigh trainer – just stop the relentless commentary please'.*

I shouldn't be bored — I have lots to do. Project number one is to digitise my LP collection and transfer them to my *iPod*. To the left of my Mac is a turntable, now gathering dust as a large paperweight. To the right is a VHS machine. Project number two is to digitise some videocassettes and convert them to DVDs. To the side lays a sketchpad and four new pencils. Annie has been reading some of my verses (yet another project) and suggests I illustrate them: 2B or HB? That is the question.

To tell the truth I'm a bit intimidated by it all. I've lost confidence. Cancer does that — it saps your will as well as your strength. And I've not even started on the boxes of 35mm slides I planned to squirt into the computer. Or all the new songs I'm supposed to learn. Trouble is, I find it hard to concentrate for more than a few minutes at a time.

I'm convinced that one of the things that's getting me down, perhaps even slowing my recovery, is my diet. I've never noticed before but fatty things like butter, cheese, chips, crisps, eggs, pies, pizzas, buns and so on are almost uniformly yellow in colour. Or at least they're drawn from the yellow part of the colour wheel. I miss the greens, reds and purples.

I tell this to the Bag Lady and nag her about getting a timetable for the bag to be removed:

Bag Lady: *'What would you like to eat?'*

Me: *'Roasted Mediterranean vegetables (red and yellow peppers, courgettes, aubergine, garlic and red onions) topped off with chickpeas, spinach and Feta cheese.'*

Bag Lady: *'You can have the Feta.'* She's not unsympathetic.

I had assumed that the reversal of the ileostomy would be straightforward — something a surgeon could do during coffee break. But it turns out to be a two-stage process. I'd only ever considered one — the first. The join in my large bowel has to be tested for leaks (we don't go into 'how' at this stage — there's only so much I can take in at one time). Assuming this is OK, we can go ahead. I knew this much.

But there's not only the join itself to consider — there's the state of the rest of the plumbing. The join may be leak-proof but if the bowel has 'suffered trauma' during the original surgery it may not work properly. The large bowel not only processes all the foodstuffs I like — it acts as a reservoir or storage facility. I've lost about a third of it and it's this ability to store waste that may no longer work. And it's not something that can really be determined until I'm out in the world bag-less. I may run back — as many do apparently — begging for a colostomy. *Noooooooooooo*. She sees the look on my face; *'if you can manage an ileostomy, you'll find a colostomy a piece of cake'.* Hmm. I might even get to eat the cake.

In one of my trips upstairs to my 'attic' I had considered the possibility that the join might not work and I'd be faced with a colostomy, so I was half-prepared for this. But I'd dismissed the idea partly because they'd given it a thorough going over when I was in intensive care (trying to get rid of the fallout from the faecal peritonitis) and partly because I simply want to believe it will not leak. The reservoir bit comes as a complete surprise and knocks me back.

I write some verses about cancer — pretty bleak stuff. I'm reminded of an interview with Richard Thompson (writer of incredibly dark, but great, songs) in which the interviewer assumes that in order to write about such despair the author must have suffered from depression or dark thoughts. *'No,'* says Thompson *'you just have to know what it feels like.'* I like this answer. It speaks to me. Feeling sad is normal and is not the same as depression. I know I'll get past this.

The Grand Union Canal passes the back of our house. I force a shuffle along the towpath for a bit of afternoon sun. Something catches my eye, a flash of turquoise. And there it is, beating down the canal towards me, a Kingfisher. I stop for the fly-past. What a treat. You can't get that on the NHS.

The Bag Lady will call the consultant to set the process for reversal in motion. It won't happen before the New Year – I have to get over this latest surgery first. While I wait for news I have time on my hands. So, LP or VHS? Or something new that I've not yet thought of? In the meantime:

Zoos

I never did like Zoos much
the thought of all them cages
I saw a polar bear once
pace to and fro for ages

I swore I'd never go again
prefer to watch on telly
they're free to roam the wilderness
and it is not as smelly

Hi, I've only read two of your recent posts as someone sent me the links. When you said that cancer can be a very lonely disease I saw your point exactly. I have felt like that on too many occasions since my own diagnosis in 2004. Recently, I worked something out. I have this overwhelming suffocating fear at times. I have the fear of reoccurrence, of the cancer taking me sooner than I ever imagined, of dying 'young', of leaving behind my husband of two years and of suffering and becoming incapable of functioning physically and communicating. I also fear that whatever plans I have strived to make for a future AFTER this nightmare, will be ruined when they tell me 'we think it's back'. So – I worked out that the FEAR is actually as destructive and threatening as the disease itself, and is in fact a whole other disease. I am trying so hard to lessen its grip on me but feel it keeps a tight grip and stops me from breaking free. I wondered also if these feelings I have would also be considered by specialists as me being 'depressed'. Or is it just part of the course of this torturous disease. I feel it breaks your heart, then eventually breaks everyone else's around you. Just wanted to share that with you.

Sarah
27th Novermber 2007

Pleased that you seem to be returning to some form of normality Ian, you are a fortunate man. I may not continue to read your blogs any more as my father is dying. You know I said he has the same as yourself, well he's had an infection that has made him terribly weak and not strong enough for any more treatment, they said that it would kill him. His cancer has spread through his lymph system too I think, due to tumours growing after the last cycle of treatment and not being able to get back on it now. He is at home now with Mum arranging his funeral etc., etc. What a remarkable man my father is. I am at a loss now, so terribly frightened scared for Dad and myself, what will I ever do without him? I am still his little girl and he wished me 'Happy

Birthday Little Girl' on Sunday and I wept, the last time I would ever hear him say that to me. You have to keep fighting this thing Ian, be one of the few that buck the trend and go on living:-)

Best Wishes, Cath
28th November 2007

Good luck Ian – keep up your cheerful spirit! I had bowel cancer in 2003 and consequently have a permanent illeostomy – can't be reversed because of radiotherapy damage – so I'm officially a bag lady!! It does get depressing – hard to explain to others – although there are people around who want to help – sometimes you feel you really are on your own – I'm due for an op in the new year to remove a bit of my lung and then I'm told I shall be fit again! It's a long hard struggle – but I find ways of distracting myself – gardening is great therapy – growing vegetables, etc.!!! Walking the dog – it all helps, I find I cannot concentrate for long – sometimes I think my brain needs attention as well – I've been told by several doctors that this is normal in cancer patients – in a way the brain seems to shut down in some way as a form of self protection and the depression one feels is almost like post traumatic stress, it does wear off eventually! Keep smiling.

Rosie
12th December 2006

My special day
December 16th 2006

It's my special day. Annie has a bottle of bubbly and some party poppers. I've been a cancer survivor for exactly one year (I've adopted the Lance Armstrong timescale for calculating these things – we regard ourselves as survivors from the time we are diagnosed rather than when we are given the all-clear). December 16th 2005 is not a date I'll forget. My emotions have been all over the place – I've had a good blub from time to time and at others have experienced waves of deep happiness and elation. Was it me or the drugs? A bit of both I guess.

Over the past 12 months I've learnt the following:

- That people are amazing
- That cancer is promiscuous – lavishing unwanted attention on not just those with the disease, but also infecting loved ones, friends and family (including dogs)
- That it's not choosy about who it goes after
- That it has side-effects which are not mentioned in the books, leaflets or consultations
- That positive thinking is hard work
- That grieving is not only normal, but good and essential to the healing process
- That it's OK for me to talk about death, but uncomfortable for others
- That an ileostomy is a right pain
- That it's OK to eat the skin of a baked potato
- That people who surreptitiously feel around the front of their trousers/skirts when in public are not necessarily perverts – they may be checking to see if their bag needs emptying
- That just sitting in the garden with a cup of coffee is a much under-rated pleasure
- And that no matter how bad I feel, there are people having a worse time than me.

Perhaps the most significant thing I've learnt is that cancer is not one, but two diseases – or rather, a disease in two parts. It's a bit like being caught up in a major disaster like the Blitz of 1940 or the Asian Tsunami of 2004. The initial response is a fight for basic survival; finding shelter, food, dealing with casualties and so on. Then, when it's all over, dealing with the aftermath.

At the risk of milking the analogy, the body is like a Thai beach or London after a night-time air raid. During the first stage we are so preoccupied that we may fail to appreciate the scale of the devastation. That only comes when the initial onslaught is over and we have a chance to look around. It may take a while for what has happened to sink in before we can move on to the next stage – rebuilding lives as well as infrastructure. But as we try to do this we are left with the inevitable question – will the bombers/sea come back?

Treatment (surgery, chemo, radio) is only part of the process of dealing with this disease. It tackles the first stage (the physical effects). There are also emotional consequences that have to be acknowledged and treated, although just how this happens seems to be a bit hit and miss.

A survey published on the BBC Health website[15] earlier this year revealed the following: 49% of cancer patients reported feeling depressed; 26% felt abandoned by the healthcare system following treatment; 45% reported that the emotional consequences were harder to deal with than the physical consequences.

I take comfort in these stats. I'm aware that my writing has taken a darker, less positive, turn of late and I had begun to think it was me. But it's not – it's this disease. I've become aware that I'm moving into the second stage – dealing with the aftermath.

There's a line in the film *Shadowlands* that goes something like *'We read to prove we're not alone'.* I write to prove I'm not alone. This blog has turned out to be a key part of my recovery, particularly as I deal with the emotional fallout. I know it has made uncomfortable reading for some people, but I want to be able to look back in five years' time and see just how far I've come. How long did it take to get through it? What did it feel like? Did I tackle it the right way? Could I, or others, have done things differently? And, more importantly, did the cancer come back? The answers to these questions may be useful to others as well. So here's my first 'end of term' report.

There are times when I feel as if I've lost a year of my life. So many plans put on hold or compromised – minor ones as well as the big ideas. It's often the small things that seem more significant – like not bothering to plant spring bulbs this year. I've had to give up my dog, work and making music (OK, I managed a few gigs, but it's not the same thing). My previously undisputed role as King of DIY has been usurped by Sister Sledge (Hammer) and her offspring. My workshop now has girlie things in it. Life used to be simple (in the grand scheme of things); now it's a series of 'what-if' scenarios.

The really cruel thing about this disease is its unpredictability. The Bag Lady once said that those she expected to survive, often don't – and those she expected not to, often do. And she's seen thousands of patients. If it confounds the professionals is it any wonder it confounds us? So I'm learning to live with uncertainty. But what does uncertainty really mean? It's more than simply wondering if the cancer might come back at some time in the future. It's about numbers, probabilities and kitchen appliances.

Some more numbers (and letters): The cancer in my bowel is classed as a *Dukes B* – it's grown into the muscle wall of the bowel but not into the lymph system. But, as it also turned up in the liver my consultant says it's technically a *Dukes D*. Just to confuse things, not all doctors use the term *'Dukes D'*. Some call it *Advanced Bowel Cancer*, meaning it's moved from the primary site into a secondary one.

Then survival rates; this is where it gets tricky. I email Cancer Research UK for the latest figures. The five-year survival rate after diagnosis for *Dukes B* is 64%. Which is pretty good. The five-year survival rate for *Dukes D* is 3%. That's right: 3%. Which is not. There is clearly a lot more between B and D than the letter 'C'. This is scary stuff and I try to up the odds. If ever there was a time to be a 'glass half full person' it's now.

It arrived at the liver via the blood stream rather than the lymph system, so that's good (or rather, not as bad). There was only one tumour on the liver – good again. So the odds are improving. What else? I help old ladies across the street and am kind to animals. I worry about the homeless and am thinking about installing solar power. Does that help?

The numbers tend to focus on the physical – the bits you can see and measure. Lifestyle must have an effect, but is not really quantifiable as far as I can tell. I'm middle aged, middle class and middle income. Age at diagnosis helps and gets me a few more percentage points. This is more like it. I do a bit more digging around and find a five-year survival rate of between 30–40% for bowel cancer with a liver resection. That's the best I can come up with. I doodle around on the guitar for five minutes while I mull this over. I was healthy, happy and fit before I got this thing. Even though I can't find any numbers relating to this, I'm going to assume it will also make a difference. Annie's relieved. She's been worrying about the 3%. She says if we'd started at 40%, she'd still have worried but now 40 seems like 100.

If they are going to come back, most cancers do so within two years of diagnosis. So 2007 is going to be a crucial year. And now the dishwasher is old and on the blink. Do we get a new one or have the old one repaired? The thought that runs through my head is *'Would I get the use out of a new one?'* You know, if I'm wrong. Living with uncertainty is as much about the prosaic as it is about the big stuff.

I woke up the other night and found myself crying because I missed my dog. By a spooky coincidence — the sort that makes you not want to believe in coincidences (but still do) — I then discovered that he'd passed away in his sleep. It made me realise that after all this time I'm starting to grieve for what has happened to me. I'm grieving for the passing of my previous life, the things I used to do and the things I always assumed I'd do. A life not burdened by the kind of uncertainty that this disease brings. The dog was a symbol of that life.

Sometimes I look in the mirror and think; *'My poor body – what have they done to you?'* The brutality of surgery and the poison of chemo have taken their toll; the Mercedes scar, the other scar down the left side of my belly, the stoma on the right and the dead brain cells. I can see where the liver is missing. My body's a bit like an overcoat that's a couple of sizes too large. All the buttons are done up, but it doesn't hang properly — there are folds and dips that shouldn't be there, because there's room underneath (I can hear my mother saying *'He'll grow in to it'*). I found it quite revolting to begin with. I cannot imagine what it's like to lose a breast or a limb. But I grieve for the parts of my body that have had to go. They've made the ultimate sacrifice. In spite of all this I consider myself one of the lucky ones; I'm still here a year on from diagnosis. I know of people who are not.

This sense of loss (both from bits that have gone, and a life that has gone) is real, much like bereavement. Whether we lose something external and obvious or an internal organ, our image of ourselves is changed. It's a bit like losing a partner (whether by death or divorce) after years of being together – we are defined by that relationship. Losing a job that we've had for a long time has a similar effect. We are no longer who we think we are.

All the books say that grieving is a natural process, hard-wired into our psyche, and an essential part of the healing process. Just how it works I'm not sure. What I do know is that 'pulling myself together' or adopting a 'stiff upper lip' and other clichés based around macho posturing don't really work (for me at least). There's a risk that if we deny ourselves, we deny other people.

For years my father refused to accept that he was ill – it was his way of coping and not giving in. He was admired for his strength and courage. All fine and dandy for him, but it left me a confused teenager and my mother a physical and emotional wreck. I came home from school one day to find her in the kitchen sobbing and systematically smashing plates. My father just sat quietly in his wheelchair. I went to stop her. *'Leave her be'.* Probably the wisest thing he said. I can understand my father's fear. But accepting that we are ill and that things are going to change does not mean giving up or resigning ourselves to fate. Acceptance (ie., grieving) and positive thinking are not mutually exclusive.

So I guess grieving has something to do with recognising and accepting our own emotional response to this disease; that there is no shame or guilt in feeling sad, helpless or alone. We can't be happy all the time. And if we can't understand how it affects us, how will we understand the affect it has on others? I've had a number of emails since starting this blog from people who have relatives with cancer who cannot or will not talk about what is happening to them. This reluctance denies loved ones a chance to grieve as well as the patient themselves.

In the end there is no right way or wrong way of coping; we each have to find our own path through all this, but I don't believe we can do it on our own. And I certainly don't believe we can do it by pretending we're OK when we're not.

For all this talk of loss, I've gained a lot as well, and I think I've ended the year slightly ahead. I've learnt so much about myself and other people. I'm much stronger (mentally) than I thought I was. My faith in myself has been sorely tested, but my determination to beat this thing has not faltered. I cannot ever imagine giving up. But positive thinking is hard to sustain, and it's been harder to summon up these past few months. The pain or discomfort (both physical and mental) is relentless – almost daily since January. I'm tired of, and bored with, cancer now.

I never imagined I'd cope with a bag. But I have – in my own way. I'm not entirely comfortable with it and will never accept it. I always seem to want to put off changing it. But once I've done it I wonder what all the fuss was about. In many ways it's changed my life more than the cancer has. Well, not so much the bag as the ileostomy. This was something I was not, and could not have been, prepared for.

It determines what I eat and where I go. I feel like a prisoner out on parole but with some sort of tag. It has more power over my life than it deserves or is entitled to. Sometimes it'll fill within half an hour of emptying – a nuisance at home, but a potential nightmare away from it, as if it's reminding me who's boss. I know there are other people who deal with this much better than I do, who live a 'free and full life' according to the leaflets. The thing that the leaflets always miss out is that we are all individuals – we respond metabolically and emotionally in different ways. Like I said earlier – there is no right way or wrong way of coping. I know my comfort zone with this thing. But like all oppressive regimes, there are periods of rebellion and risk-taking. I'm going through one right now. Last week I ate a baked potato – *with skin* – and last night I had a curry. If I leave this entry half completed, you'll know that this was a risk too far.

My core beliefs have not changed, but my view of the world, the way I see things, has become more polarised over the year – a little less grey and a bit more black and white. As a result I've become less tolerant – particularly of people who get worked up about the trivial things in life and seem to ignore the important issues. I realise that this is grossly unfair and it does bother me. Sometimes it's extremely difficult to distinguish between the trivial and the important. All I can say is that one night in a hospital bed listening to someone in distress, sorts out what really matters and what does not.

When I was in intensive care I went through some sort of Pauline conversion – a wave of calm came over me and I resolved that if I got out of there, I would be a different person. I would no longer let the things that used to bother me, do so. No more cursing people on their mobile phones while driving, no more shouting *'I don't believe it'* at the television – I would become a model of sweet reasonableness. Like all resolutions it lasted a few weeks. But I'm not going to beat myself up about it. Life's too short – which is probably why I'll never buy a cookery book by Heston Blumenthal.

I am however, careful not to confuse the trivial with the simple. My faith in the simple is stronger than ever. Sitting in the garden with a cup of fresh coffee, or riding my bike with my best gal by my side are not things I take for granted.

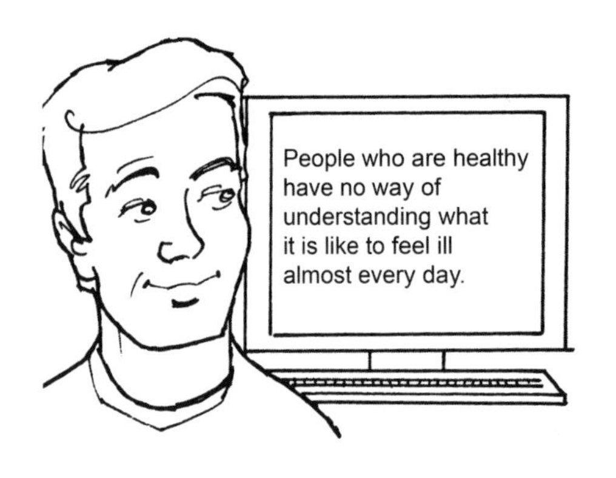

I've been very lucky – I could not have got through this without the love and support of all my friends – or the complete strangers who've taken the time to email or leave a comment on my blog. This disease, or rather its side effects, have made me grumpy, sad, irrational and unreasonable – and through all this Annie has never complained. Well she has a bit, but not much. She's been disappointed that our life together has been put on hold and she's been through the fears and anxieties that I've experienced, as well as a few of her own. But she's never once flinched from supporting me. She really would give me her last *Rolo*.

My good friends Bob and Margaret (from Nebraska) sent me a copy of a book[16] written by their doctor, John S. Campbell, himself suffering from chronic illness. He writes:

'People who are healthy have no way of understanding what it is like to feel ill almost every day'.

I'm sure most people can empathise with someone who is seriously ill – it's the everyday bit that is so hard to explain or imagine in a way that other people could possibly understand. Particularly with cancer, when for so much of the time we appear 'normal' on the outside.

In the course of treating patients as well as dealing with his own condition, the good doctor observes that healthy people often avoid the sick – and the sick often push the healthy away. There have been times when I've not wanted to see other people and I know some people have found it difficult to see me. Interestingly these instances have not coincided. I felt at my lowest during chemo – it poisoned my brain as well as my body. I know others found it hard to cope with the physical change I underwent when in hospital for the bowel op. My fear was being seen as a mental wreck – theirs was dealing with a physical wreck. That didn't stop them caring though.

When I first became ill I knew communication would become important. By that I mean the dialogue that passes between the patient and doctors. They know we look up stuff on the internet; some are able to take that into account when dealing with us. I do believe the medical profession is making a real effort to communicate and, on the whole, I have few complaints. One doctor insisted on addressing me when answering Annie's questions, but most were inclusive.

What I had not realised all those months ago is how important communication between those with the disease and their loved ones would be. Forget *'sorry'* – the hardest word to say is *'death'*. It's not something that drops easily into conversation:

'By the way, you decide about the dishwasher – I won't be here.'

or

'I've booked two tickets to Switzerland – one single and one return'.

Yet it's something that is always on the mind of the cancer survivor. JJ posted the following quote a little while ago:
'I did not die there, but I came close, and there was a moment,

perhaps there were several moments, when I tasted death, when I saw myself dead. There is no cure for such an encounter. Once it happens, it goes on happening; you live with it for the rest of your life.'[17]

It's impossible to unthink these thoughts once you've had them, and it's difficult to explain what it feels like to other people. It's not that they come up every day, they just catch you out from time to time, when you're least expecting it.

The point where communication is in most danger of breaking down is when patient and loved ones want different things. When, for example, the patient wants to decrease or stop aggressive therapies and the family wants them to continue. The family is angry, hurt and frightened because they see their loved one as 'giving up', while the patient is saying; *'I can't take this pain anymore'.* There were times when I didn't want to go back to chemo. I knew I had to – I wouldn't be able to have liver surgery without it. But some days Annie had to (metaphorically) push me out of the door. I can understand if someone feels they've had enough.

Annie and I are starting, tentatively, to talk about these issues. Not everyday and not in any great detail. Just enough so it doesn't catch us unawares. It's understandably harder for her than me but is easier done when I'm feeling fit and well and we're both happy, than later should the cancer return. There's a tension in all this – how much to say? She's the one person who really needs to know – and indeed wants to know – what I'm thinking. But at the same time I want to protect her, to keep some stuff back. In the end we agree that I'll tell her everything, no matter how difficult.

I've never really been scared of death *per se* – but of late the process bothers me. I say this as someone who has had to confront his own mortality and is, frankly, a little scared at the prospect of dying. I wish for a painless and dignified end (and who wouldn't?). As I said in an earlier blog, I'd prefer to expire quickly and quietly at the age of 96 having just come off stage at Glastonbury. Although at 96 we'll probably be playing in an old folks home or will have cornered the cruise ship market.

Cancer in general, and hospital in particular, has forced me to take a hard look at what happens to people, especially the elderly, when they become ill. And it's not great. Older people are not always treated with the respect or dignity they deserve when they become ill, even by the well-intentioned. This is not something new. Cicero, writing some 2000 years ago:

'Old age will only be respected if it fights for itself, maintains its rights, avoids dependence on anyone, and asserts control over its own to its last breath.'[18]

So, in a way he might never have imagined, we're taking Cicero's advice by turning the spare room into a gym. I need to get fit to recover from the past year – and then get even fitter for the years ahead. I do not want to become ill when I'm old and end up in hospital again. While it might just possibly be a place for a painless end, dignity flies out the window once you lie in that particular bed.

In this past year I've come across a lot of metaphors and analogies for describing the process of living with cancer. Most involve journeys of one form or another. I've also heard a lot about fighting this disease; indeed it's a phrase I've used often enough myself. But I realise that for me at least it is not appropriate. I'm a coward at heart and my response is to run rather than stay and fight as such. I have my own analogy.

I'm in a car on a long straight road. This car runs on will power and my foot is pressed hard to the floor as I try to outrun the cancer. Every so often I glance in the rear-view mirror and see that it's getting closer. The car won't go any faster so I have to jettison something to lighten the load. First to go is the bowel and I open up a gap. But slowly and surely it catches up. I throw out the liver and again put some distance between us. Only this time I can't – daren't look back. Not yet anyway. I'm not ready. I grip the wheel tightly and lean forward – as if this could possibly make any difference to my speed. The car is hurtling along with the radio playing *'Born to run'* by Bruce Springsteen at full blast.

And that's it. Time alone will tell how this plays out. I have my own preferred ending; we come to a fork in the road, I go one way, the cancer goes the other. I glance out of the window and see the cancer looking at me, frustrated as our paths diverge. I resist the temptation to stick two fingers up just in case the road doubles back. But it doesn't and I settle back to enjoy the ride. Our paths never cross again. My choice of which way to go comes down to luck, nothing more and nothing less.

The idea of marking, celebrating even, this special day is important – a bit like birthdays, but with added poignancy. This has been such an eventful year – probably the most eventful of my life so far. From the moment the fateful words were uttered, life was changed forever. There are times when this disease, or rather its effects, have brought me to my knees. At other times I've felt a sense of exhilaration – from the feeling that if I can deal with this I can deal with anything.

Finally – a touch of *déjà-vu*. I've seen a couple of TV programmes recently about choirs, one featuring a group of 80–90-year-olds in the USA[19] singing songs by The Clash and Jimi Hendrix and another featuring a UK choir singing the big choral works: Mozart, Verdi, Handel, etc. I mention to Annie that I'd like to join a choir (can't read music, but that's never stopped me before). I really need to engage more with my creative side – in his book, Campbell talks a lot about the role of creativity in healing; *'Creativity is the best path to making lemonade out of lemons'.*

I tell Annie that I'll make enquiries after Christmas and see what opportunities there might be. She looks up and I can tell she's excited; *'You're back to where you were last year'.* I'm puzzled. I'd forgotten, but she's right. I'd been thinking, in the latter part of 2005, that I'd like to join a choir – even got in touch with one. But I'd abandoned the idea last December. Can I really be trotting down this same old road again?

I'm thankful to be here and I will get the flags out. And if my liver is up to it, I'll raise a glass – for myself, and everyone else affected by this wretched disease: to those who've got me this far; to those who continue to survive; and for those who do not. We are all part of the Cancer Family.

'But since it falls unto my lot
That I should go and you should not
I'll gently rise and softly call
Goodnight and joy be with you all.'

(from) *The Parting Glass* traditional folk song

Ian, thank you for posting this. Your special day is also a special day for me also. It is my second wedding anniversary today. I got married three months after my treatment finished. I cried through the whole day. I was heartbroken for myself and my life. My brother came and stood behind me with his hands on my shoulders to give me support and strength I needed saying my vows. On January 12th 2007 it will be three years since my diagnosis. Like you I do not feel that I am ready to go yet. I have much still to do. I had a scare recently and I felt the nearness of the fear again and so close to the wheels of treatment all over again. But – I am 'normal' according to the tests and I am relishing that state of being! Ian – you have much still to do yourself. Keep posting and look forwards when you can. A very merry Christmas to you and yours and may the coming year bring you increasing health and happiness.

Maria
16th December 2006

Maria, my best wishes to you and your hubby on your wedding anniversary. The support that your brother has given you seems a very poignant gesture to me … perhaps he was offering to shoulder some of that burden of pain you were carrying?? I am thinking of how hard I sometimes find it to ask for support, or to take it when it is offered … not wanting to infect others with my fears. I shall be anticipating January 12th with you, and raise a glass to you and all those I have come to know. Take care.

Ian, I struggled to find the right words when it was my own anniversary … 'celebrate' somehow was wrong for me. It was more that I wanted the significance of the day and of the time since that day to be acknowledged, witnessed??? Maybe I am wrong to even search for words, falling into that trap of thinking there are 'right words'. Tonight I will raise my glass and think of coming to know you in the last few months, with my best wishes for you both in my heart.
I am reminded of a favourite post from another forum whereby people requested to join 'le Club dangereuse'. The only criterion for entry was, (naturally), a claim to have carried out a dangerous act. Examples for those who have undergone breast surgery might include … wet shaving of the axilla, wearing a wired bra, carrying a weight greater than 5kg, gardening, having false nails applied, having blood taken or an injection into one's 'bad' arm … etc., etc.
From your post I can see that you have actually two claims for membership and wish to recommend your immediate entry.

My very best wishes to you both, JJ
17th December 2006

I've never commented on your blog before and I kinda don't know what to say but I just wanted you to know that I'm so proud of you for everything that's happened and how you've got through it all so positively and with such brilliant humour. You've made me laugh even through all the serious bits! I can't wait for you to get your appointment and get the operation done so you can crack on in the snazzy gym! It was soooo lovely to see you over Xmas and thanks for all your help on my big dissertation (which got handed in fine). I wish I got to see you more and I love you so much. You're the best step dad ever and always will be.

Helen xxx
16th January 2007

Well, before you know it Ian, summer will be here and the Bag Lady will be no more! I really wish you well, I am routing for you every step of the way (you know why). Your life will never be as it was, we all know that, but you'll begin to get back some of the person you were as time progresses, you'll adjust to being 'normal' again. You and your family have had a tremendous amount of stress to cope with (I know) it changes you all but your clock is about start ticking again – 2007 will be a good year for you:-)

As always, love Cath
21st January 2007

[15] BBC News online (Health) April 4th 2006.
[16] *A Journey: Creative Grieving and Healing*; John S. Campbell, M.D. 2006.
[17] *The New York Trilogy*; Paul Auster, Faber & Faber, 1987.
[18] in *A Journey: Creative Grieving and Healing*; John S. Campbell, M.D. 2006.
[19] *Young@Heart*; http://www.youngatheartchorus.com/

Epilogue

February 2nd 2007

'We have to take care of your cancer.'

Hmm. So, strictly speaking I still have cancer.

'There may be cancer cells present which were smaller than the resolution of the scanner last time we looked ... we hope that they will have been mopped up by chemotherapy.'

I'm in Oxford. A new consultant. He says he's met me before but I don't remember. He's very nice and helpful. I tell him that I still have numb toes and he promises to follow this up with the anaesthetist who did the operation.

The 'take care of' is an odd phrase. At first I thought he meant 'take care of' as in look after. Then driving home I pondered on something more sinister – 'take care of' as in eliminate/get rid off? A simple enough phrase yet two conflicting meanings. A BBC survey reporting on communication between doctors and patients reveals that if a doctor says *'your tumour is progressing'* around half of patients think that it's a good sign[20]. Doctors and patients; two peoples with a common tongue divided by a common language.

I'm on my own; Annie is still trying to impress quadratic equations on unwilling minds. She's experimenting with a new pedagogy – the *'You can listen to your iPod later'* approach to learning. I miss her – she's my slip catcher – I usually only take in half of what is said to me and we compare notes when we get home. So I have to listen very hard today. Luckily the consultant is patient. Annie's missing out doubly – there are new cranes on site. I have to provide as much feedback about these as I do the consultation: *'Did you watch them from the tea shop?'* (As a matter of fact I did).

I have two coffees this morning so I'm a bit sparky and alert. I take most of it in. I'll have a scan in two months (which would be six months after the operation) to see if there are any unwanted visitors.

Bowel cancer cells do not play fair – they cheat – they play dead in order to fool the chemo drugs and wake up when they've gone. I'll have another scan six months after that. I'm sent for a blood test before I leave; I'll have one each time I come to Oxford from now on. *'Why? What does the blood test indicate?'* Sorry Annie – forgot to ask.

That was last week – a pleasant drive, sun shining, The Eagles at full volume in the car and the prospect of a relaxing chat with the consultant among the dreaming spires of Morse country. Today I'm back in cow country (concrete that is) with a tube up my backside. I'm told the rich and famous pay good money to have this done to them. Good grief. If I were that rich, I'd pay someone to have it for me.

It's such a contrast; there is no dignity with bowel cancer – at some point it involves lying prone while tubes, lights, cameras, fingers even, rummage around places that are usually off the beaten track – all the time under the watchful eyes of a critical audience. You'd think with all the prying, cameras, lighting and discussion afterwards, that the cancer cells would have had enough – *'I'm a tumour – get me out of here'.* Channel 4 is missing a trick. *This* is Reality TV.

On the other hand, a tumour on the liver is much more civilised and up market. Even the resulting wound is called the Mercedes Scar.

But no amount of fancy names or euphemisms can disguise the fact that cancer is a poxy disease. Two people I've come to know well through this blog have lost loved ones in the past few weeks. There are times when I feel guilty about (apparently) getting better when others aren't – although I know this is not what these *e-friends* would want. In their darkest moments they still have time and generosity of spirit to encourage my recovery.

The band will be playing at a fund-raiser for a children's cancer charity in a few weeks' time. I'm keen to do it – but the organisers and some of the people in the audience have lost children to this disease and I don't know how to approach it. *'Is everyone having a good time? Let me hear you say yeah'* hardly seems appropriate. Yet the cancer community is amazingly resilient – stoical even. Everyone acknowledges there are people having a worse time than them, no matter how bad they themselves might feel.

I ponder on this as the tube goes in:

'I'll just check to see if they left any staples in first.'

Staples? Left? Any?

'It looks OK.'

I'm still thinking about the implications of this when they shove it in further. **JEEZ** – I'd forgotten what this was like.

'I guess you haven't used those muscles in a while.'

My insides get a fresh coat of paint. I hope one coat is enough. Then compressed air to spray it all around. The first images don't show much so they pump some more. So much that the bag inflates. This is gross. Luckily I put a clean one on this morning. If it flies off ... ileostomy *piñata* anyone?

The radiologist thinks the join has healed and there are no leaks. She turns the video monitor round for me to see. Looks a bit like Channel 5 late on a stormy night. A doctor is called to check the images. He smiles and puts his hand on my shoulder; *'I think we can put you back together'*.

We can put you back together.

There was a time when I thought I'd never hear these words (or words like them). Is this really the beginning of the end? Somehow it seems to carry more weight than if he'd said *'You no longer have cancer'*.

JJ emailed to say it sounds like something from the *Bionic Man*. I can just see it – *The Man with the Bionic Bowel*. I'll be played by Donald Sutherland[21], Annie (prim school teacher by day, feisty crane operator by night) will be played by Meg Ryan[22] and Lester, my faithful ex-dog, will be played by Rowdy[23], the stuffed canine hero from *Scrubs*.

Nuts and seeds will hold no fear for the *Man with the Bionic Bowel*. A couple of drops of *Extra-Virgin 3-in-1* lube once a week to prevent rust in winter and seizure in summer and life will be hunky dory. I just don't want it designed by Sir Richard Rodgers – I don't want all the pipe work on the outside of my body. Although I could make a feature of it I suppose.

After 14 months or so I can really start to look forward to the bag coming off. 2006 has been a pig of a year. 2007, on the other hand is the Year of the Pig, as was the year in which I was born. It turns out I am a *Fire Boar*. According to *Wikipedia*, this is a good thing, it does not mean a tiresome person whose only interest in life is combustion.

2007 is going to be my year – *The Comeback Kid*. I'm hoping that the bag reversal will be done and dusted by the summer. It's going to be a busy one; my step-daughter Helen graduates from Uni, I have a BIG birthday (the one where you get free eye tests, the Winter Fuel Allowance and a B&Q Diamond (geezer) Card) and Annie and I would desperately love a holiday. So – lots to think about and plans to make. In the meantime, the Bag Lady will discuss the results of the scan with the consultant.

I'm not going to worry now about whether or not the bionic bowel will work. The join does not leak and that's the main thing. The bag can come off and the ileostomy can be reversed. If I end up needing a permanent colostomy – well that's something I'll deal with when the time comes. Just as long as I can get one in carbon fibre. Flesh-tone is *so* last year.

Then – as I write these last few words, and with the sort of timing we'd get if this really was a TV show – a message from the Bag Lady: *'it's all systems go'.*

I am back in my home briefly before 'My sister's Big Day' next Wednesday. Your latest update was just what I needed and made me chuckle – and sympathise. I had colorectal surgery nearly two years ago, one to ensure that 'the uninvited guest' had not taken up residence and to repair damage done by an over enthusiastic 'practitioner'. When doing the sigmoidoscopy in OPD – he obviously thought that he was working for that well known drainage clearance company and also forgot that I was not under anaesthetic or a cadaver!!! I never cease to wonder what makes someone want to deal with the waste department of our digestive system – and to delve in regions, dark and mysterious. Thank God they do – for our sake. What a journey you have made and are still making. You special and incredible bod. I recently spotted a Meccano set offered for sale and wondered if Annie might like to build a crane all of her own!!!!! Bless you both – keep writing.

Barbara
4th February 2007

[20] BBC News Online (Health) November 15th 2005.
[21] Suggested by Nicola Picola.
[22] A fantasy of Annie's that I've only just discovered.
[23] This was my late dog's dearest wish.

One more thing

Hindsight is a wonderful thing. It can also be dangerous – or at the very least confusing. I've forgotten what the pain was like. And I know I have some more pain to come. So would I do anything differently if I were to be diagnosed now, instead of December 2005? I suppose I could have bought some bigger trousers earlier. And taken ear defenders into hospital sooner.

This is a hard one; looking back I think I handled it the best way I could – for me. Not only that, I can *only* change those things that are within my direct control – and I would guess that with cancer at least 90% of what happens is beyond us.

One of the best decisions I made, once I knew I had cancer, was to tell people about it and to tell as many as I could. I know some people are reluctant, perhaps through fear or embarrassment, to say anything. But I wanted to shout it from the rooftops – or rather email as saying the words out loud was just too difficult at that stage. I wanted to say *'I'm scared, but I'm going to beat this thing. Help me'.* And people did.

One of the clever tricks, if you can master it, is to read just the right amount of information. Too little and you can be lost or left behind by what the medics have to tell you. Too much and you can scare yourself witless. Needless to say, 'just the right amount' is a very personal thing. So listen to the voice inside your head if it's telling you 'enough is enough'.

If I were to offer just one piece of advice it would be this: go and see your doctor if you get the squits for more than a couple of days. You have to get to the bottom of the problem. Better to waste a GP's time than waste a life.

Appendix: Still crazy after all these fears

The effects of disease on the mind – and vice versa – have been written about at length, as have the effects of drugs on creativity. But it's not until you experience it at first hand that it begins to sink in that something deep and magical is happening.

Early on in my treatment I experienced bizarre hallucinations, most probably due to the effects of morphine. Coleridge is reputed to have written much of the *Ancient Mariner* in a very short period of time, while under the influence of opium. While not claiming to be a Coleridge, I too experienced a 'mind dump' of verses during November 2006 in the aftermath of liver surgery. They arrived in my head, quite unannounced, over about a two-week period – and then stopped as quickly as they had come. Most arrived fully formed, only needing the odd word changing here and there. I cannot recall any obvious stimulus. Indeed the subject matter varies greatly, so it's unlikely that any one trigger could have provided the vital spark.

Campbell writes convincingly about the role of creativity as a means of coping with, and recovering from, illness. I take him to mean 'creativity' in its broadest sense, from the literal – painting and writing as therapy – to the more general – perhaps finding unusual and inventive solutions for coping.

I thought at the time that it might be some kind of defence mechanism – the brain's equivalent of putting its hands over its ears when faced with the enormity of bringing the body back from the edge. Nothing since then has happened to make me change that view. Pity – it was fun while it lasted.

Whatever the explanation – and there undoubtedly is a good scientific explanation – disease does seem to play hard and fast with the mind. I mention all this in case it happens to you; I just want to provide some reassurance that you're not barking.

Cancer and the Battle of Little Big Horn

Cancer does what cancer wants
A selfish gene indeed
Whizzes through the body
At supersonic speed

Never takes a prisoner
Leaves the dead behind
Starts inside the body
Infiltrates the mind

I seem to live a halfway life
Between the dead and living
I take from those around me
And hope they keep on giving

It makes me oh so fearful
I think only the worst
If it decides to kill me
I want to get in first

And then I'd thwart its evil plan
Like Sitting Bull did Custer
But that would take more courage
Than I could ever muster

I'd love to be a dancer

I'd love to be a dancer
I like to dance a lot
In *the* days of King Arthur
I'd be Sir Prance-a-lot
I envy all the dancers
They always get the girl
I long to take her in my arms
And give my love a twirl

The only time I'm confident
Is when I've had a drink
I had a go at tap-dancing
But fell into the sink

I envy all the dancers
The way they move with ease
It's hard to be that graceful
When you've got dodgy knees

Internet love

He sat at his computer
"My dearest, darling, Pet"
he was writing to a woman
whom he had never met

he was 'male, non-smoker'
keen on art and books
she was 'female, sporty'
neither cared for looks

at least that's what they told themselves
as they prepared to meet
he with folded newspaper
a sign he hoped discreet

she brought her computer –
a laptop – just in case
the pixels on her hard drive
looked nothing like his face

he settled for a cheesy scone
she a soda-pop
it took a while before they spoke
and then they didn't stop

they talked about their families
and things they meant to do
dreams and aspirations
things better done by two

cards were on the table
romance was in the air
each picked up a lonely heart
found themselves a pair

My dog is like a red, red rose

My dog is like a red, red rose
His smell is over-powering
His ancestors cannot be Wolf
He sees a cat – he's cowering

He's such a fussy eater
I have to feed by hand
His ears flop in his water bowl
I tie them with a band

He cannot chase a rubber ball
Won't even fetch a stick
The only thing he's mastered
Is a disappearing trick

He will not win a major prize
Though he has looks a plenty
I fear his brain is just too small
Either that or empty

In spite of this I love him
He's my dog, after all
Though he is on the small side
And I am on the tall

Sunday morning

I wish we'd made love this morning
I was feeling in the mood
Nothing too exotic, mind
And certainly not rude

But you were wanting breakfast
"I've to get up" you said
I'd have settled for tea and toast
And a nice warm cuddle instead

"I've got to put the washing on
And polyfill the ceiling
I've got no time for all that lark
– but don't let go that feeling"

So off you go, my busy love
And I pull the covers tight
If not this Sunday morning
Then maybe Sunday night

The alligator and the alli-baiter

The alli-baiter grabbed a stick
And poked and laughed till he was sick
Suddenly a mighty splash
Tormentor gone within a flash
He shows his head – a toothy grin
And hand and foot stuck to his chin
Parents wail in deep despair
"our lad would never harm the hair…
only ever brought us pleasure
till that gator got his measure"
The lesson for the naughty boy?
An alligator's not a toy
But flesh and blood and animal cunning
If you should see one – best start running

Zoos

I never did like Zoos much
the thought of all them cages
I saw a polar bear once
pace to and fro for ages

I swore I'd never go again
prefer to watch on telly
they're free to roam the wilderness
and it is not as smelly

Benny

Benny was a boxer
And a rubbish one at that
In 30 fights he'd won just once
The rest he'd been knocked flat

He'd shuffle and he'd wobble
And dance like he was pissed
Till his chin fulfilled its destiny
With his opponent's fist

He thought he'd make the big time
And be a star on telly
But you can't be a winner
With legs that work like jelly

So now he opens village fêtes
Garden Centres and the like
And instead of swanky limousines
He goes home on his bike

The other fifth Beatle

The Beatles were my favourite
When I was of that age
Each LP (that's long player)
Cost half my weekly wage

Carefully on the Dansette
Anticipate the song
"And tonight on broomstick ..."
Then I'd sing along

I always wanted to be John
Rarely one of the others
(and when I wasn't being him
– I'd be the Ev'ley Brothers)

I found the broomstick easier
To play than my guitar
And 'cos I didn't practice much
I didn't get that far
I'd have a go at 'Three Blind Mice'
But two chords weren't enough
For 'Lady Madonna'
And all their other stuff

It wasn't till my Forties
I finally found a way
To buy myself a real guitar
Cost half my monthly pay

Months and months of practice
Anticipate the day
'Hang on guys I'm coming'
But they've since gone away

Sources of information

There's a lot of information out there. Possibly too much. Some of it is good, some of it is bad and some is so so. Here's a list of websites, articles and books that I've found helpful, in one way or another.

Useful websites

http://www.bowelcanceruk.org.uk/factskeystats.htm
http://www.cancerhelp.org.uk
http://www.maggiescentres.org
http://www.macmillan.org.uk
http://www.dansac.co.uk
http://www.fittleworth.net
http://www.dignityindying.org.uk/
http://www.livestrong.org
http://www.bowelcancer.tv
http://www.cctrust.org.uk

Articles

http://www.cctrust.org.uk/article3.htm
http://www.cctrust.org.uk/article5.htm
http://www.bbc.co.uk/health/tv_and_radio/how_to_have_a_good_death/index.shtml
http://news.bbc.co.uk/1/hi/health/4435208.stm
http://www.dailymail.co.uk/pages/live/articles/health/healthmain.html?in_article_id=406955&in_page_id=1774

Books

Alda, Alan, *Never have your dog stuffed*. (London: Arrow Books, 2007)
Not a cancer book, but a good description of an end-to-end anastomosis in Chapter 20. And an enjoyable diversion from cancer books.

Armstrong, Lance, *It's not about the bike: my journey back to life* (London: Yellow Jersey Press, 2001)
A grim but inspiring account of testicular cancer by the man who came back to win seven *Tours de France*.

Bennett, Alan, *An average size rock cake: in Untold Stories* (London: Faber and Faber, 2005)
A reassuring description of bowel cancer – it gave me heart.

Campbell, John S., *A Journey: creative grieving and healing* (New York: iUniverse, 2006)
Chronic disease from the point of view of a doctor who is also the patient.

Marchetto, Marisa Acocella, *Cancer Vixen* (London: Fourth Estate, 2007)
Breast Cancer as strip cartoon; an alternative and very creative way of describing how the disease affected the author and those around her.